Malnutrition

Edited by Muhammad Imran and Ali Imran

Published in London, United Kingdom

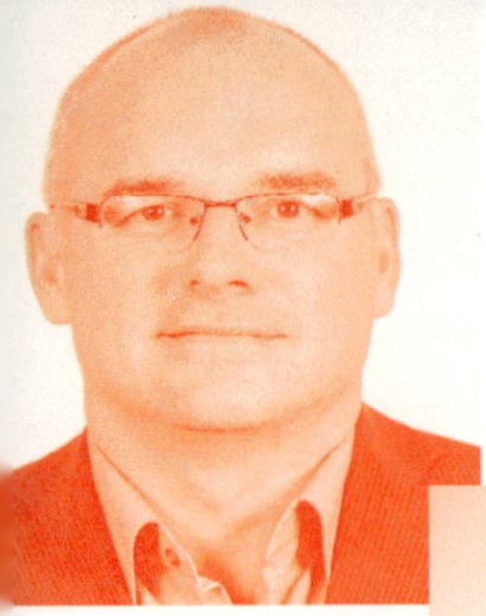
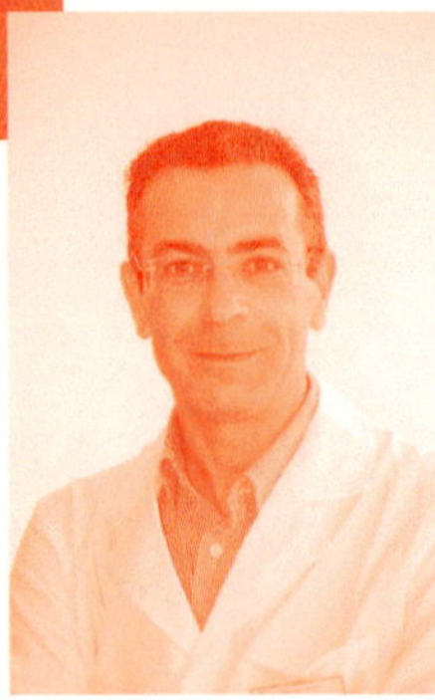
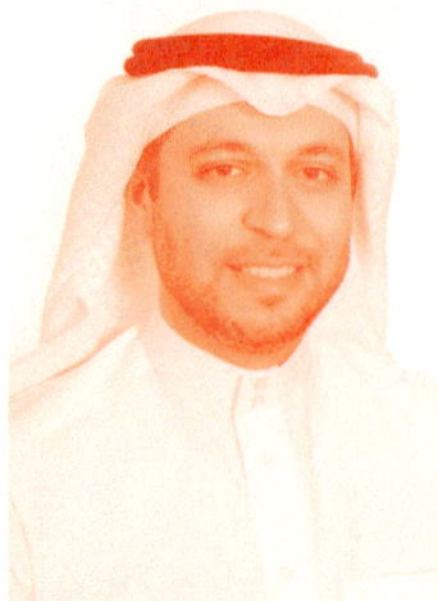
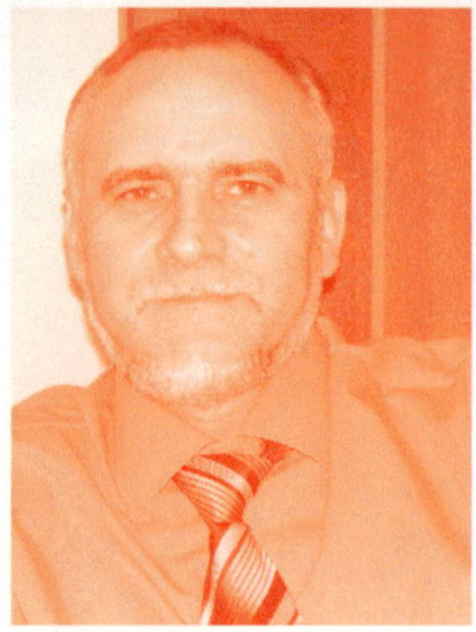
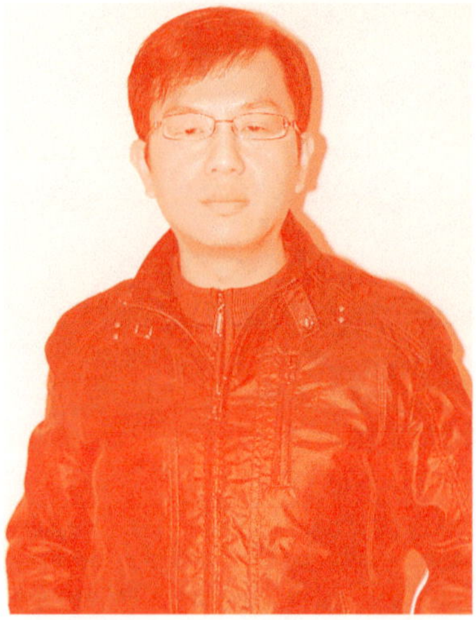
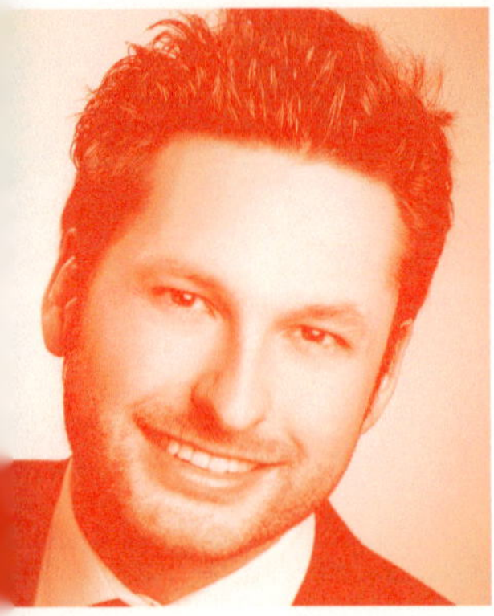
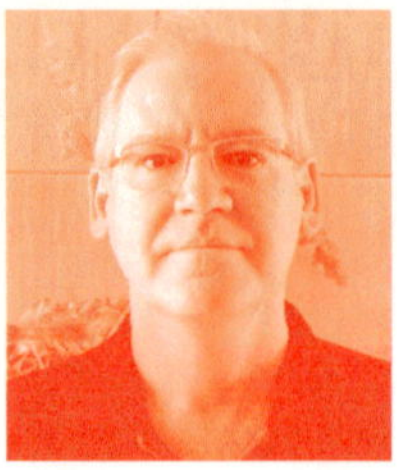

IntechOpen

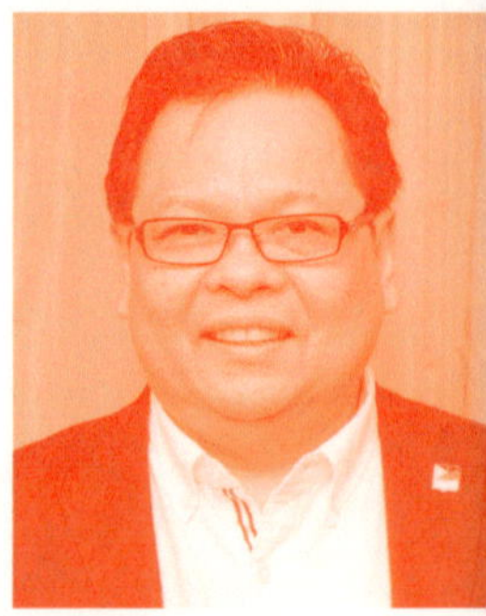
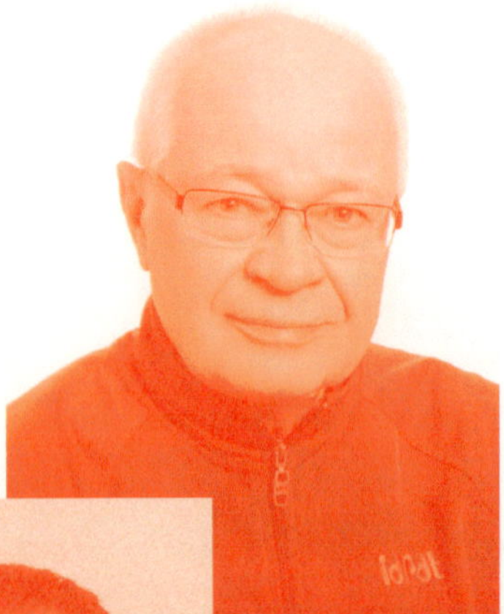
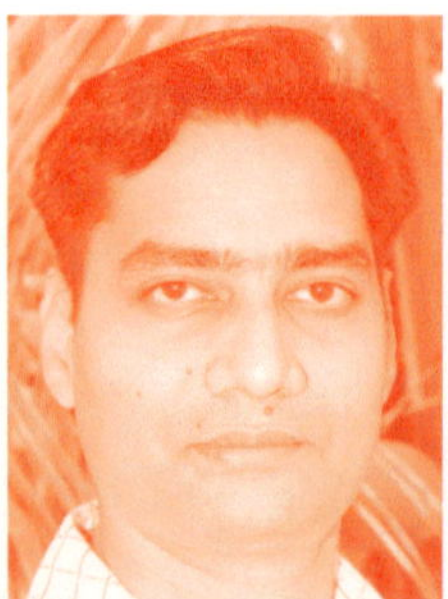
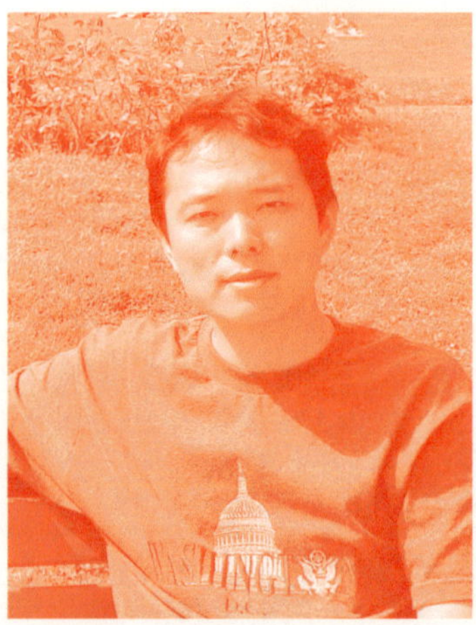
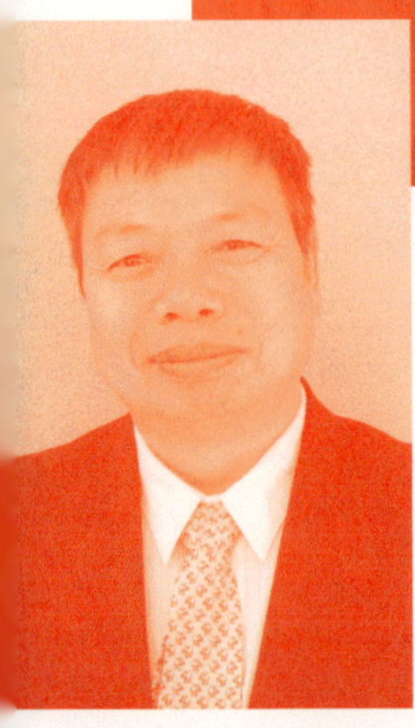
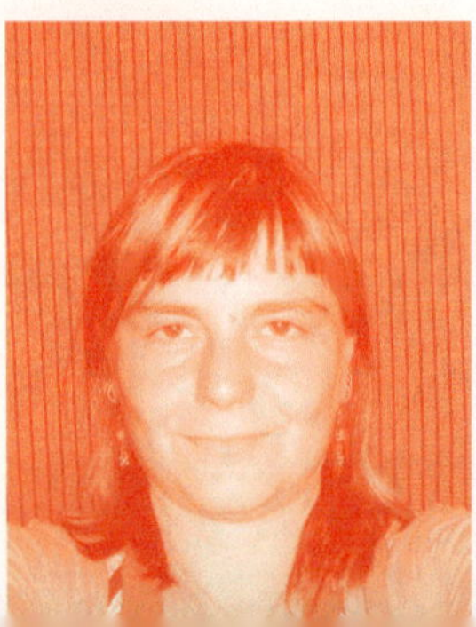

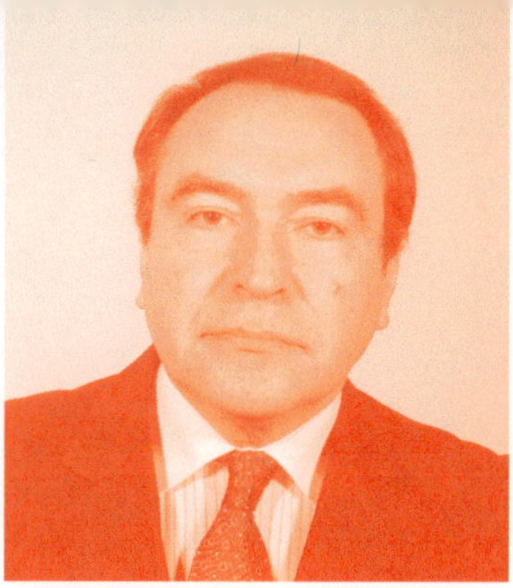
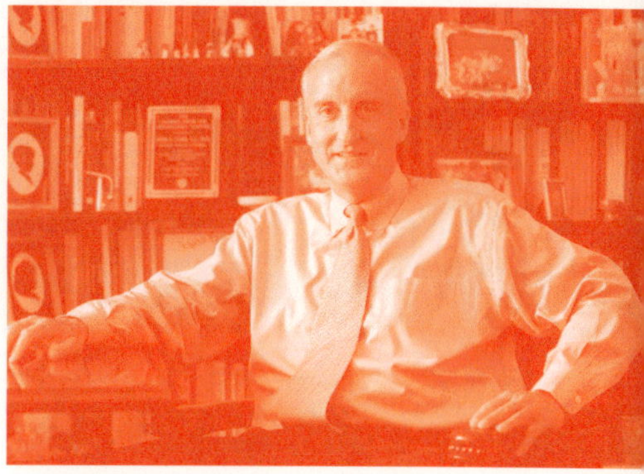
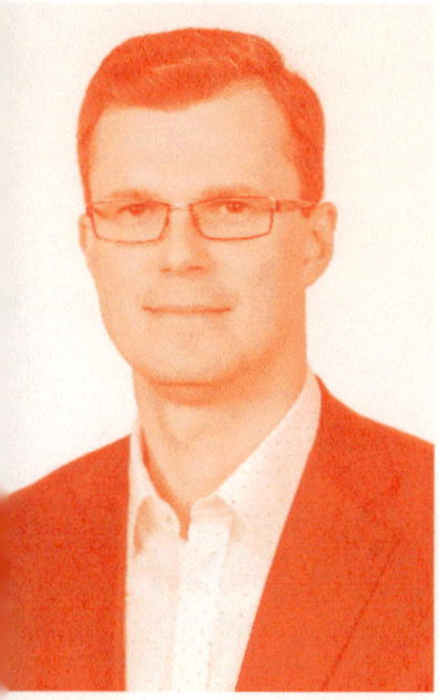
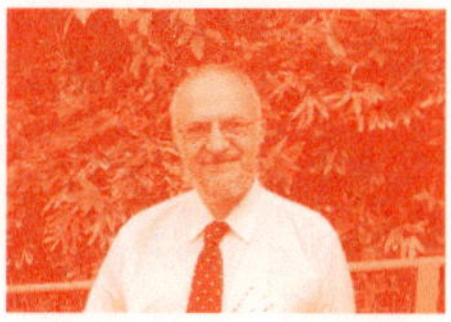
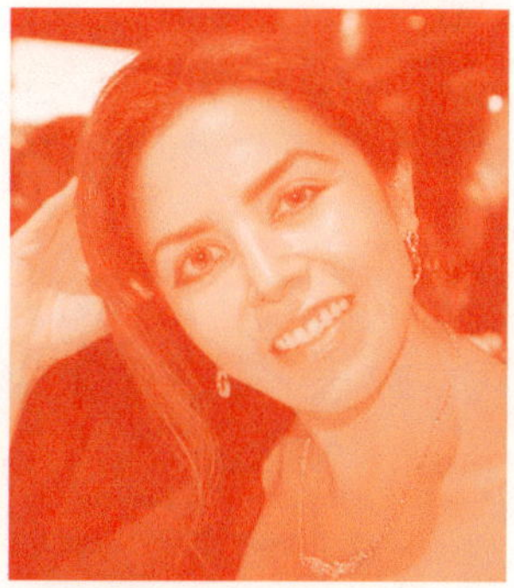

Supporting open minds since 2005

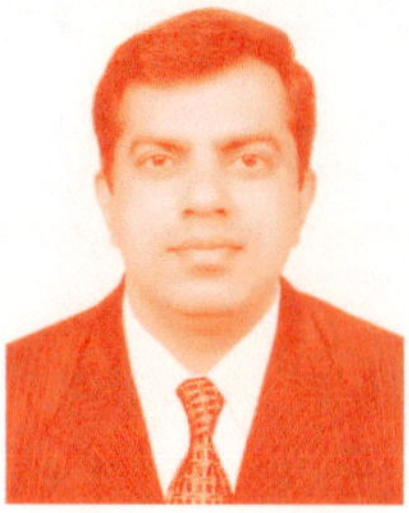
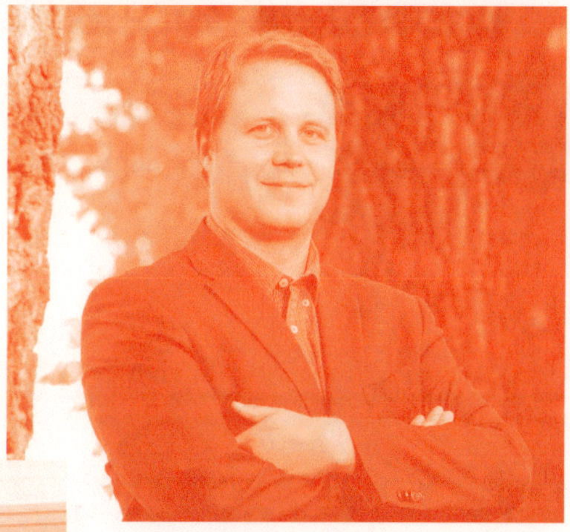
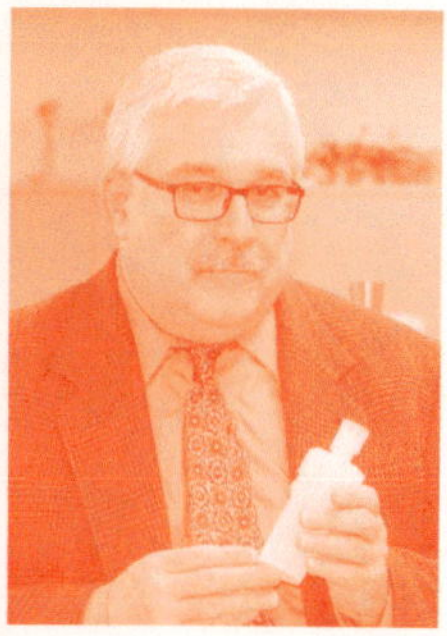
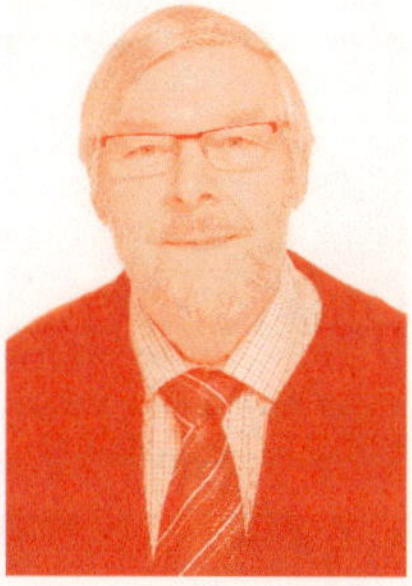
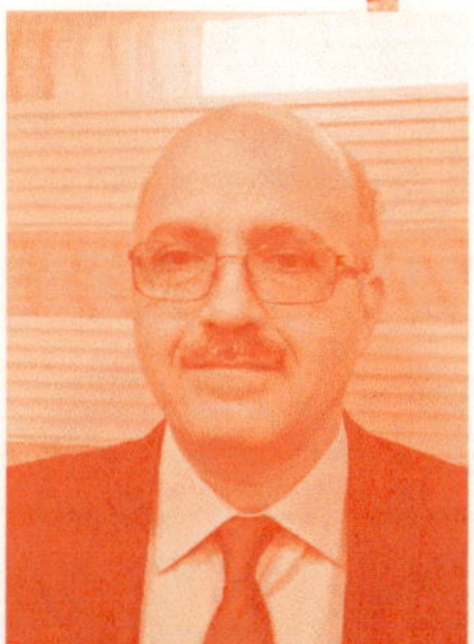
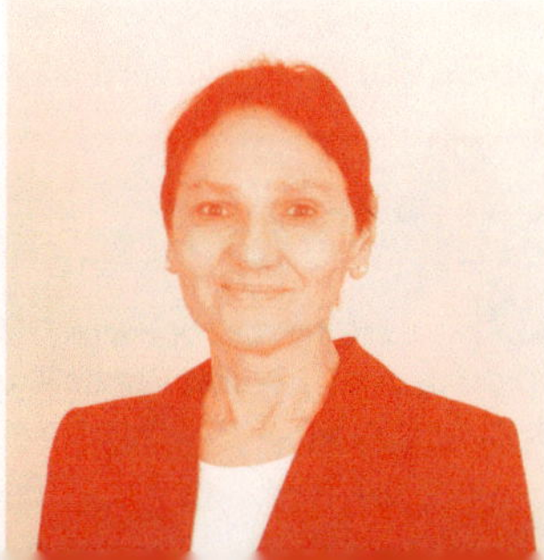
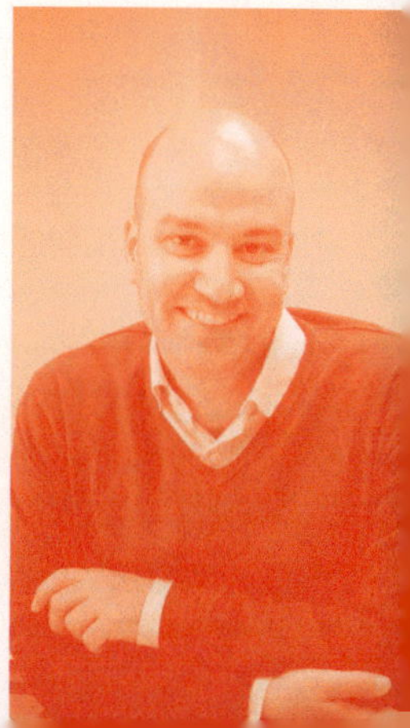

Malnutrition
http://dx.doi.org/10.5772/intechopen.77861
Edited by Muhammad Imran and Ali Imran

Contributors
Francisco Javier Ros Forteza, Natisha Dukhi, Joseph Choge, Mohanad Mousa Kareem, Majid S. Jabir, Junsheng Huo, Chunhong Zhang, Kathleen Hefferon, Muhammad Imran Farhan Saeed, Tabussam Tufail, Ali Imran

First published in London, United Kingdom, 2020 by IntechOpen
IntechOpen is the global imprint of INTECHOPEN LIMITED, registered in England and Wales, registration number: 11086078, 5 Princes Gate Court, London, SW7 2QJ, United Kingdom
Printed in Croatia

British Library Cataloguing-in-Publication Data
A catalogue record for this book is available from the British Library

Additional hard and PDF copies can be obtained from orders@intechopen.com

Malnutrition
Edited by Muhammad Imran and Ali Imran
p. cm.
Print ISBN 978-1-83880-516-6
Online ISBN 978-1-83880-517-3
eBook (PDF) ISBN 978-1-83969-156-0

Meet the editors

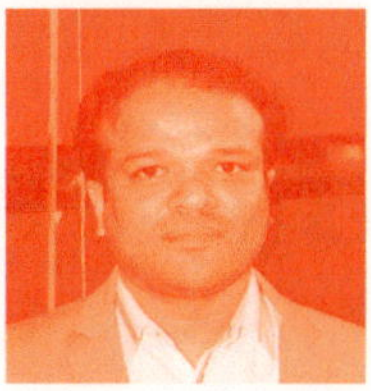

Dr. Muhammad Imran received his Ph. D from the University of Agriculture, Faisalabad in 2013 with distinction. His research interests are the preparation of cost-effective polyphenol based dietary interventions against metabolic syndromes and conversion of agro-waste materials into value-added products along with expertise in functional and nutraceuticals foods. He has more than 85 publications in impacted international and national journals with a cumulative impact factor of more than 200. He has also published 11 book chapters with international publishers such as Springer and Elsevier. Moreover, he is also working as section head of a Research Unit and has produced more than 14 M. Phil students within his research area. He has also served as a guest editor for international journals.

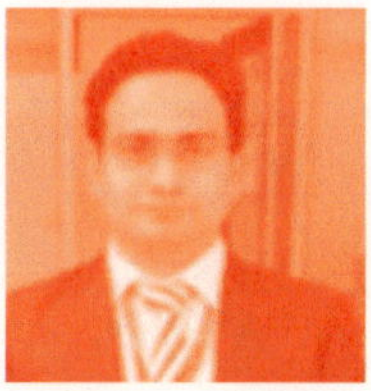

Dr. Ali Imran (Associate Editor) earned his Ph. D from the Agriculture University, Faisalabad in 2013 with distinction. His research expertise includes the formulation of the cost-effective polyphenol-based dietary interventions against human maladies. Being a researcher, he has published more than 50 articles in high impact international journals with a cumulative impact factor of more than 80. Further, he has also published 7 book chapters with international publishers. He is also working as an academic editor in Hindawi groups in the Journal of Biomedical Research International. He has assisted two Ph. Ds and 12 MPhil students within his research domain. He is also working as the section in charge in his HI TEC laboratory.

Contents

Preface **XI**

Section 1
Introduction to Malnutrition **1**

Chapter 1 **3**
Introductory Chapter: Malnutrition
by Farhan Saeed, Muhammad Imran, Tabussam Tufail and Ali Imran

Chapter 2 **9**
Biofortification of Crops Using Biotechnology to Alleviate Malnutrition
by Kathleen Hefferon

Chapter 3 **21**
Vitamins
by Mohanad Mousa Kareem and Majid S. Jabir

Chapter 4 **39**
Malnutrition: Current Challenges and Future Perspectives
by Joseph Kiprop Choge

Section 2
Malnutrition and Global Determinats **65**

Chapter 5 **67**
Wernicke Encephalopathy in Elderly Related to Severe Malnutrition
by Francisco Javier Ros Forteza

Chapter 6 **81**
Global Prevalence of Malnutrition: Evidence from Literature
by Natisha Dukhi

Chapter 7 **97**
Detection of Nutrient-Related SNP to Reveal Individual Malnutrition Risk
by Junsheng Huo and Chunhong Zhang

Preface

This edited volume is a collection of reviewed and relevant research chapters concerning the developments within the malnutrition field of study.

This book covers a very relevant topic that not only proved a major disaster for developing economies but also caused problems in developed economies. Malnutrition causes severe structural and functional abnormalities that hinder the growth of the individual, but also society in general. This book provide complete insight into the problem, pathophysiology, impact and rectifying strategies.

Each contribution comes as a separate chapter complete in itself but directly related to the book's topics and objectives.

The book is composed of two sections: 1.) Introduction to Malnutrition, and 2.) Malnutrition and Global Determinants.

The "Introduction to Malnutrition" includes the following chapters: "Introductory Chapter: Malnutrition", "Biofortification of Crops Using Biotechnology to Alleviate Malnutrition", "Vitamins" and "Malnutrition: Current Challenges and Future Perspectives". The second section, "Malnutrition and Global Determinants", includes the following chapters: "Wernicke Encephalopathy in Elderly Related to Severe Malnutrition", "Global Prevalence of Malnutrition: Evidence from Literature" and "Detection of Nutrient-Related SNP to Reveal Individual Malnutrition Risk".

The target audience comprises scholars and specialists in the field. This book will provide deep insights into the problem, pathophysiology and tackling strategies.

Muhammad Imran
University of Lahore,
Pakistan

Ali Imran
Government College University,
Pakistan

Section 1

Introduction to Malnutrition

Chapter 1

Introductory Chapter: Malnutrition

Farhan Saeed, Muhammad Imran, Tabussam Tufail and Ali Imran

1. Introduction

Malnutrition is defined as not having enough food to eat or more than feeling hungry. Insufficient intake of calories (a measure of energy the body needs), protein (necessary to build muscle and to keep the body healthy), iron (for appropriate blood cell function) as well as different types of nutrients can cause malnutrition [1]. In a person's intake of energy as well as nutrient imbalances, excesses or deficiencies are referred to as malnutrition. Two broad groups of conditions are covered by the term malnutrition. One is 'undernutrition' which comprises micronutrient deficiencies or insufficiencies (a lack of significant vitamins and minerals), underweight (low weight for age), wasting (low weight for height), as well as stunting (low height for age) [2].

Among the children fundamental cause of mortality and morbidity is malnutrition [3]. Approximately half of the mortality in children attributed to undernutrition around the globe [4]. In children's mental and physical development, it poses a risk as well that is result in deprived academic accomplishment [5]. To ensure in early childhood intellectual development, proper physical and a strong immune system adequate nutrition is indispensable [6, 7]. In the world under the age of five 110 million (19%) are moderately or severely underweight and 170 million (30%) of children are moderately or severely stunted [8]. In Asia reside approximately half of all stunned children, under five years of age children 51 million (8%) are wasted, as well as in Asia live two thirds of all wasted children [9]. The dynamic prospective of the society, socioeconomic development of children and future health affects by malnutrition. Prevalence of child malnutrition compared to other developing counties Pakistan has been reported to have one of the highest levels [10]. About 50% were anemic, 44% were stunted, 33% were anemic (iron deficiency), 33%of all children were underweight, 15% are wasted, According to the National Nutrition Survey. In Pakistan compared to other developing countries in the prevalence of child malnutrition there has been a little reduction, In the last two decades [11]. In less developed countries a major public health and social problem, childhood malnutrition still remains, despite economic and social development [12, 13]. In childhood malnutrition the contributing factors are infectious diseases, vaccination, poor sanitation, food insecurity, household socioeconomic status, birth spacing, parity, micronutrient intake, lack of proper knowledge of nutrition, maternal education, inappropriate complementary feeding, inadequate breast feeding and exclusive breastfeeding as well as low birth weight. In the world the Pakistan is among the countries with the highest rates of child malnutrition, as well as than in other South Asian countries its progress and health in child nutrition remains slower.

2. Undernutrition

If undernutrition occurs before two years of age or during pregnancy, it may result in permanent problems with mental and physical development. Known as starvation, the extreme undernourishment, may have symptoms that comprise swollen legs and abdomen, very poor energy levels, thin body and a short height. Frequently cold and infections too often get people. On the micronutrient that is lacking depend the symptoms of micronutrient deficiencies. Not enough high-quality food being available to eat most often undernourishment is because of it. Most often related to poverty as well as high food prices. Be short of breastfeeding might contribute as might a number of infectious diseases for instance measles, malaria, pneumonia as well as gastroenteritis which enhance nutrient requirements. Dietary deficiencies as well as protein-energy malnutrition, there are two main types of undernutrition. A lack of vitamin A, iron and iodine comprises common micronutrient deficiencies. Deficiencies may become more common, due to the body's increased need, during pregnancy. Two severe forms of Protein-energy malnutrition are kwashiorkor (a lack of just protein) and marasmus (a lack of protein and calories). Within the same communities as undernutrition is beginning to present overnutrition in the form of obesity, in some developing countries. Malnutrition other causes comprise bariatric surgery and anorexia nervosa [14].

3. Wasted and stunted

In two major ways nutritionists have categorized undernutrition, Since the 1970s. If children have a small mid-upper arm circumference and low weight for-height, to signify acute undernutrition which is taken, they are defined as wasted and in need of treatment. If children have a low height-for-age, to signify chronic undernutrition which is taken they are defined as stunted. Low weight-for-age classified children as underweight, because of stunting or wasting or both thus, undernutrition index is composite. At the population level widely used these markers to assess child undernutrition as well as who are wasted or stunted a high prevalence of children is considered a public health problem [15]. At the level of interventions and programmatic design, however, the two categories of undernutrition were approached very differently.

Wasted children contain an elevated risk of dying that by nutritional therapy may often rapidly reduced [16]. To prevent deaths associated with child wasting, making therapy available is so considered essential. On the other hand, including fetal development, over long periods children have poor growth in height they are categorized as stunted. For rapid nutritional correction is not willing this growth faltering as well as consequently rather than treatment considered to require prevention, these outcomes in terms of policy leading to the separation, programmed interventions, guidance as well as financing: at the individual level, now viewed as separate conditions acute undernutrition as well as chronic undernutrition, and among policy makers as distinct outcomes are routinely reported [17].

A new classification for malnutrition is established by John Conrad Water low. to show the stunting which results as of chronic malnutrition with height-for-age combines weight-for-height (representing acute episodes of malnutrition), rather than using just weight for age measurements, the classification established by Water low. Over the Gomez classification one advantage of the Water low classification is that even if ages are not known weight for height can be examined [18].

Degree of PEM	Stunting (%) height for age	Wasting (%) weight for height
Normal: Grade 0	>95%	>90%
Mild: Grade I	87.5–95%	80–90%
Moderate: Grade II	80–87.5%	70–80%
Severe: Grade III	<80%	<70%

The above table shows the classifications of malnutrition by WHO, with some modifications being commonly used.

4. The effects of malnutrition

More likely than others to be caught in the weakened immunity as well as downward spiral of malnutrition, people who restrict their food intakes, whether because of an eating disorder, illness, desire for weight loss, and lack of appetite. One or more of the following also susceptible: malnourished, poor, hospitalized and very young or old. When medical tests of a malnourished individual signify compromised immune system increase dramatically rate of death and sickness.

When an individual becomes malnourished, often worsens disease by malnutrition that in turn gets worse malnutrition. For disease when impaired immunity opens the way often begins a destructive cycle: when impairs appetite by disease, interferes with absorption as well as digestion, excretion increases or metabolism alter then further suffer nutrition status [19].

5. Effect of malnutrition on economy of a country

Malnutrition as well as global hunger remains big challenges in the last two decades, despite achieved significant progress. In the world about 805 million people continue to suffer as of chronic hunger and people suffer from micronutrient deficiencies more than 2 billion. Furthermore, in low and middle-income countries, obesity and overweight are on the rise.

Huge economic and social costs are imposed by hunger and malnutrition that are able to be felt at societal, household, and individual levels. For instance, according to the FAO, the global economy per year US$1.4–2.1 trillion cost for hunger and undernutrition or global gross domestic product 2–3%. To eliminate hunger and malnutrition, the economic returns are able to as well extremely elevate. From reducing child undernutrition, there are substantial, lifetime economic benefits demonstrated by evidence as of IFPRI-led research. For instance, every dollar spent on interventions in economic returns to reduce stunting is estimated to generate about US$34, in India.

Malnutrition as well as hunger is expensive. It is predictable that because of undernutrition (GDP) 2–3%, equivalent to per year US$1.4–2.1 trillion is lost and because of overnutrition annual GDP another 2–3% is lost. Collectively, because of malnutrition global GDP 5% (per year US$3.5 trillion) is lost [20].

Each dollar spent in economic benefits iodizing salt generates $30; each dollar spent in economic benefits on iron supplements for children aged six to 24 months and for mothers generates $24. Each dollar spent in economic benefits on vitamin A generates estimated to be $40 or more. To reduce chronic undernutrition need bundling micronutrient interventions for instance, individuals that decrease iron, iodine and vitamin A deficiencies with the condition of other micronutrients (for example to reduce the duration and severity of diarrhea zinc powders needed) as well as energy-dense foods. About the importance of these for healthy child growth communication with caregivers and mother is also important. Across countries the costs related with doing so differ as do the benefits however in a typical developing country, each dollar spent in economic benefits on this bundle generates around $18.

These are extraordinarily high benefit: cost ratios, by the standards of economics. Not merely that, trivially low the costs of these investments. Who are vitamin A deficient in the 95 million preschool children to eliminate vitamin A deficiency from every North American and western European less than two dollars would be enough, investment of about $650 million dollars a year an additional annual, as well combating undernutrition spent to current expenditures. Nearly two billion people are affecting by iodine deficiencies and 80 million pregnant women are affecting by anemia. Needed to reduce chronic undernutrition – for the bundle of interventions a larger investment is needed, suggest by current estimates that in the 34 countries per year around nine and half billion dollars would reach 90% of children that in the developing world account for 90% of the burden of undernutrition [21].

Author details

Farhan Saeed[1], Muhammad Imran[2], Tabussam Tufail[1] and Ali Imran[1*]

1 Institute of Home and Food Sciences, Government College University Faisalabad, Pakistan

2 Faculty of Allied Health Sciences, University Institute of Diet and Nutritional Sciences, The University of Lahore, Lahore, Pakistan

*Address all correspondence to: dr.aliimran@gcuf.edu.pk

References

[1] Torpy JM, Lynm C, Glass RM. Malnutrition in children. JAMA. 2004;**292**(5):648-648

[2] Young E. Food and Development. Abingdon, Oxon: Routledge; 2012. pp. 36-38. ISBN: 978-1-135-99941-4

[3] Bryce J, Boschi-Pinto C, Shibuya K, Black RE. WHO child health epidemiology reference group. WHO estimates of the causes of death in children. Lancet. 2005;**365**:1147-1152. [CrossRef]

[4] World Health Organization. Children: Reducing Mortality. 2017. Available from: http://www.who.int/mediacentre/factsheets/fs178/en/ [Accessed: 03 March 2018]

[5] Pelletier DL, Olson CM, Frongillo E Jr. Food insecurity, hunger, and under nutrition. In: Bowman BA, Russell RM, editors. Present Knowledge in Nutrition. 8th ed. Washington, DC, USA: ILSI Press; 2006. pp. 701-713

[6] Asad N, Mushtaq A. Malnutrition in Pakistani children, its causes, consequences and recommendations. The Journal of the Pakistan Medical Association. 2012;**62**:311. [PubMed]

[7] Ali SS, Karim N, Billoo AG, Haider SS. Association of literacy of mothers with malnutrition among children under three years of age in rural area of district Malir, Karachi. The Journal of the Pakistan Medical Association. 2005;**55**:550-553. [PubMed]

[8] Stevens GA, Finucane MM, Paciorek CJ, Flaxman SR, White RA, Donner AJ, et al. Nutrition impact model study group. Trends in mild, moderate, and severe stunting and underweight, and progress towards MDG 1 in 141 developing countries: A systematic analysis of population representative data. Lancet. 2012;**380**:824-834. [CrossRef]

[9] United Nation International Children's Emergency Fund (UNICEF). Levels and Trends in Child Malnutrition. 2014. Available from: http://www.unicef.org/media/files/Levels_and_Trends_in_Child_Mortality_2014.pdf [Accessed: 25 November 2015]

[10] Di Cesare M, Bhatti Z, Soofi SB, Fortunato L, Ezzati M, Bhutta ZA. Geographical and socioeconomic inequalities in women and children's nutritional status in Pakistan in 2011: An analysis of data from a nationally representative survey. The Lancet Global Health. 2015;**3**:e229-e239. [CrossRef]

[11] Planning Commission, Government of Pakistan, Pakistan Institute of Development Economics. National Nutrition Survey. Islamabad, Pakistan: Planning Commission, Government of Pakistan, Pakistan Institute of Development Economics; 2011

[12] Masibo PK, Makoka D. Trends and determinants of undernutrition among young Kenyan children: Kenya Demographic and Health Survey; 1993, 1998, 2003 and 2008-2009. Public Health Nutrition. 2012;**15**:1715-1727. [CrossRef] [PubMed]

[13] Pasricha SR, Biggs BA. Undernutrition among children in South and South-East Asia. Journal of Paediatrics and Child Health. 2010;**46**:497-503. [CrossRef] [PubMed]

[14] World Health Organization. What is malnutrition? [Online]. 2020. Available from: https://www.who.int/features/qa/malnutrition/en/#:~:text=Malnutrition%20refers%20to%20deficiencies%2C%20

excesses,of%20energy%20
and%2For%20nutrients [Accessed:
26 July 2020]

[15] Bergeron G, Castleman T. Program responses to acute and chronic malnutrition: Divergences and convergences. Advances in Nutrition. 2012;**3**:242-249

[16] Bhutta ZA, Berkley JA, Bandsma RHJ, et al. Severe childhood malnutrition. Nature Reviews. Disease Primers. 2017;**3**:17067

[17] Development Initiatives. 2018 Global Nutrition Report: Shining a Light to Spur Action. London: WCRF International

[18] Waterlow JC. Classification and definition of protein-calorie malnutrition. British Medical Journal. 1972;**3**(5826):566-569

[19] Finch CE. The Biology of Human Longevity: Inflammation, Nutrition, and Aging in the Evolution of Lifespans. London: Academic Press; 2007

[20] FAO. The State of Food and Agriculture. Rome: Food and Agriculture Organization of the United Nations; 2013

[21] Hoddinott J. The economic cost of malnutrition. In: The Road to Good Nutrition. India: Karger Publishers; 2013. pp. 64-73

Chapter 2

Biofortification of Crops Using Biotechnology to Alleviate Malnutrition

Kathleen Hefferon

Abstract

Malnutrition affects millions of people around the world, and the vast majority are found in developing countries. Malnutrition increases childhood mortality, amplifies poor outcomes during pregnancy, and is responsible for a variety of health disorders ranging from anemia to blindness. Biofortification of crops using biotechnological approaches such as genetic modification and genome editing holds promise as a powerful tool to combat malnutrition. This chapter describes progress that has been made in the development of biofortified staple crops to address malnutrition.

Keywords: malnutrition, biofortification, biotechnology, transgenic plant

1. Introduction

Micronutrients play a variety of roles in metabolism and homeostasis. Micronutrient deficiency, also known as malnutrition, can result in the increased incidence of many diseases and metabolic disorders. To improve nutritional status through a balanced and enriched diet, the quantification and bioavailability of vitamins and minerals must be determined. The analysis of micronutrient content can enhance nutritional quality and improve nutritional status [1].

The level and composition of micronutrients vary significantly among crop varieties. Globally, cereals, roots, and tubers represent major staple food staples. While these crops are rich in carbohydrates, they may have very low quantity or poor-quality proteins and micronutrients [2]. In Asia, people who depend on rice are more prone to vitamin A deficiencies due to the lack of this micronutrient. This in turn makes them more susceptible to a number of health problems such as blindness [3]. Similarly, over 20 different dietary minerals are considered essential for human health. Global-level deficiencies in iron (Fe), zinc (Zn), and iodine (I) are most common as they have a significant negative impact on public health.

Since the concentrations of most vitamins in the edible parts of the plants are frequently low, one research goal has been to identify biochemical pathways involved in the synthesis, translocation, and accumulation of micronutrients in plant tissues [4]. Further understanding of these mechanisms would enable us to manipulate these pathways and improve their micronutrient content through metabolic engineering [5]. Although these strategies have demonstrated some degree of success, issues such as appropriate nutrient levels, bioavailability, ready adaptation by farmers, and acceptance by consumers must be addressed [6].

For the past several years, food supplementation has been the main strategy used for vitamin and mineral fortification. This strategy has a number of weaknesses, such as the decreased bioavailability of micronutrients after food processing. Biofortification has been considered an alternative solution and can be achieved via (i) an agronomic approach, (ii) conventional plant breeding, and (iii) genetic engineering [2, 7–10]. In the following chapter, the micronutrient biofortification of edible crops by genetic engineering will be examined.

2. Uptake and bioaccumulation of minerals by plants

Minerals can accumulate in various ways and are stored in different compartments/organelles by plants species. These in turn can be affected by growing conditions as well as through interactions with other mineral nutrients [11, 12]. For example, iron is an essential element for plant metabolism, growth, and development [13]. Iron can be absorbed by the roots in the form of Fe^{2+}, then becomes oxidized to Fe^{3+}, is chelated by citrate, and then is transported to the top of the plant [14]. Zinc, another essential nutrient for plant growth and development, accumulates preferably in the vacuoles of the epidermal leaf cells as electron-dense deposits [15, 16].

3. Mineral biofortification using transgenic plants

Biofortification of crops using modern biotechnology techniques has been under exploration. Transgenic crops with increased accumulation of important minerals such as iron, zinc, and calcium within edible tissue are under development. Simultaneously, research into transgenic crops with reduced concentrations of antinutrients such as phytate has been developed. Antinutrients reduce the bioavailability of minerals by interfering with their absorption in the gut [9].

4. Transgenic crops biofortified with iron and zinc

Rice is one of the most well-studied cereals for mineral biofortification. Rice (*Oryza sativa*) is a staple of a large proportion of the world's poor and is deficient in several essential micronutrients. Transgenic rice plants have provided a model system to enhance the amount of bioavailable iron and zinc that is found in the edible seed (endosperm) of cereals. Plant scientists discovered that metal transporter proteins found in many crop species can be used for multiple metal substrates, including iron, zinc, and even cadmium. These metal substrates can be taken up from the soil and into the roots. Researchers found that loss of function mutants of these transporter proteins creates a loss of uptake of all three of these metals into plant cells [17]. Ferritin, the iron storage protein, can assist in metal accumulation in plant tissue. Masuda et al. demonstrated an increase in accumulation of ferritin as well as an increase in iron translocation via the overexpression of the iron (II)-nicotianamine transporter OsYSL2 within rice endosperm. Transgenic lines generated higher levels of both iron (6-fold in the greenhouse and 4.4-fold in the paddy) and zinc (1.6-times), demonstrating that introduction of multiple genes involved in iron and zinc homeostasis could improve iron biofortification more than the introduction of a single gene. Later, Masuda et al. [18] increased iron and zinc accumulation through increased iron uptake and transport using the ferric iron chelator, mugineic acid. Transgenic plants that were generated expressed the ferritin gene from soybean (SoyferH2), and are driven by two endosperm-specific promoters, in addition to the barley nicotianamine synthase gene (HvNAS1), two nicotianamine aminotransferase genes (HvNAAT-A and HvNAAT-B), and a mugineic acid synthase gene (IDS3) (to increase mugineic acid production in rice plants). These transgenic plants were tolerant of iron-deficient soil and displayed increased iron accumulation by 2.5-fold. Under iron-sufficient conditions, transgenic rice lines increased iron accumulation by 4-fold as much as lines that had been cultivated in either commercially supplied soil (iron-sufficient conditions) or calcareous soil (iron-deficient conditions). Transgenic lines expressing both ferritin and mugineic acid biosynthetic genes displayed signs of iron-deficiency tolerance in calcareous soil, and the iron concentration in polished T3 seeds increased by 4 and 2.5 times, respectively, compared to nontransgenic lines grown in normal and calcareous soil. Recently, Li et al. [19] have identified a zinc transporter protein family (ZIP) for taking up divalent cations in plants. The researchers found that by overexpressing the ZmZIP5 protein, iron and zinc levels were increased in seeds of rice plants. Similarly, Beasley et al. [20] constitutively expressed the rice (*Oryza sativa* L.) nicotianamine synthase 2 (OsNAS2) gene in bread wheat. This brought about the upregulation of nicotianamine (NA) and 2′-deoxymugineic acid (DMA), which are important for iron and zinc transport and nutrition. Transgenic plants accumulated higher concentrations of Fe and Zn in wheat grain endosperm and iron bioavailability was increased in white flour milled from field-grown CE-OsNAS2 grain.

There are other ways for iron deficiency to be addressed using transgenic plants. For example, Sharma and Yeh [21] used an ethyl methanesulfonate (EMS) mutant in *Arabidopsis* that is tolerant of iron-deficient soil and demonstrated the accumulation of 4–7 times higher amounts of iron than wild type in roots, shoots, and seeds. This mutant presented a dominant "Metina" phenotype that constitutively activates the Fe regulatory pathway by optimizing Fe homeostasis and thus may be useful in Fe biofortification. Similarly, Qiao et al. [22] found that the wheat gene encoding the cell number regulator (CNR) protein showed enhanced tolerance to Zn, and overexpression of *TaCNR5* in *Arabidopsis* increased Cd, Zn, and Mn translocation from roots to shoots. This indicates that heavy metal tolerance characteristics can be used as a tool to biofortify cereal grains with micronutrients.

Since the same molecular machinery is utilized for transporting iron and zinc into plants, increasing iron content in rice also brings about increased zinc accumulation. As an example, Aung et al. [23] generated a transgenic line of rice commonly eaten by consumers in Myanmar, where approximately 70% of the populace is iron deficient. This line overexpressed the nicotianamine synthase gene HvNAS1 to enhance iron transport, the Fe(II)-nicotianamine transporter gene OsYSL2 to transport iron to the endosperm and the Fe storage protein gene SoyferH2 to increase iron accumulation in the endosperm. The rice plants were shown to accumulate over 3.4-fold higher iron concentrations, in addition to 1.3-fold higher zinc concentrations compared to conventional, nontransgenic rice. The results of this study indicate that transgenic rice biofortified for increased iron content could address both iron as well as zinc micronutrient deficiency in the Myanmar population.

Paul et al. [24] generated transgenic high-yielding indica rice that expressed the soybean-derived ferritin gene. Transgenic plants produced over 2.6-fold higher levels of ferritin than their nontransgenic counterparts, even in the fourth generation of rice plants. Upon milling, transgenic rice grains provided 2.54-fold and 1.54-fold increases in iron and zinc content, respectively. Similarly, the iron transporter gene MxIRT1 taken from apple trees was utilized by Tan et al. (2015) to generate transgenic rice plants that exhibited an increase in iron and zinc of threefold, in addition to a decrease in cadmium concentration. Cadmium is thought to compete with iron and zinc for transport and accumulation in the rice endosperm and, thus, lower levels of cadmium to reduce toxicity in the rice seed.

Improvements in iron and zinc biofortification have also taken place using other approaches. Trijatmiko et al. [25] demonstrated that plants expressing rice nicotianamine synthase (OsNAS2) and soybean ferritin (SferH-1) genes possessed enriched endosperm Fe and Zn content. A Caco-2 cellular assay illustrated that increased iron and zinc levels found in these rice plants were bioavailable. Transgenic plants generated by Banakar et al. [26] expressed high levels of nicotianamine and 2′-deoxymugenic acid (DMA). These plants were able to accumulate up to 4-fold more iron and 2-fold more zinc in rice endosperm, in addition to lower levels of cadmium compared to wild-type plants.

Other crop species have also been studied for iron and zinc biofortification using biotechnology. Tan et al. [27] improved iron levels in the pulse crop chickpea (*Cicer arietinum* L.) by increasing iron transport and storage through a combination of chickpea nicotianamine synthase 2 (CaNAS2) and soybean (*Glycine max*) ferritin (GmFER) genes. Transgenic chickpea plants that overexpressed these genes illustrated a doubling of NA concentration, suggesting an increase in iron bioavailability. Pearl millet was examined by Manwaring et al. [28] for iron and zinc biofortification by improving the currently available gene pool. High iron and zinc-biofortified pearl millet would be advantageous for poor regions of the world where soil management or supplementation programs are ineffectual. Narayanan et al. [29] have expressed the iron sequestering Arabidopsis AtVIT1 gene in cassava plants to increase iron storage in the crop's roots. Iron concentration also increased in stem tissues and accumulated in plant cellular vacuoles.

5. Calcium-biofortified transgenic plants

The calcium content of crops can also be increased using biotechnology. These advances hinge on improved knowledge of how soluble calcium ions found in the soil are transported and accumulate in plant tissue [30]. Calcium plays a significant role in general cell signaling; how calcium transporters are expressed can thus influence a plant's ability to withstand stress, ward off pathogens, and can influence the nutritional status of animals and humans. Park et al. [31] have generated transgenic tomato, potato, lettuce, and carrots expressing high levels of calcium transporters. One of these calcium transporters, known as a short cation exchanger (sCAX1), can increase calcium transport into plant cell vacuoles [32]. Enhanced calcium absorption has been demonstrated in animal models that were fed transgenic carrots. Similarly, Sharma et al. have examined the potential of finger millet, an orphan crop with high calcium content, by studying the mechanisms behind calcium uptake, transport, and accumulation in grain. It has been reported that climate change may act detrimentally on mineral accumulation in different crop species; this could limit their further availability from food crops for both humans and animals [33].

6. Bioaccumulation of vitamins in plants

Vitamins such as β-carotene and folic acid are critical for human health. The development of microbial biochemistry facilitated the understanding of the biosynthetic pathways involved in vitamin production in plants. All vitamins that are required in the diet are synthesized by plants with the exception of ascorbic acid (vitamin C), which is specifically synthesized by eukaryotic cells [5, 34, 35]. Often biosynthesis is compartmentalized within various organelles. With greater comprehension of the metabolic pathways involved in vitamin production, plants can be developed with high levels of vitamin accumulation.

7. Vitamins and transgenic biofortification strategies of edible crops

GM technology also has the potential to reduce the global burden of malnutrition and hidden hunger. Vitamin- or mineral-enriched GM foods (GM biofortified foods) are considered to be the next generation of GMOs. Non-GM biofortified crops have been widely developed and commercialized, but the applied conventional breeding techniques may be inadequate for crops with a low level or absence of a certain micronutrient [36]. A recent review has summarized successful R&D efforts in the field of GMOs with increased micronutrient content in staple crops [37].

8. Vitamin-biofortified rice

The well-known example of GM vitamin biofortification is Golden Rice, enriched with pro-vitamin A (β-carotene) [38, 39], followed by vitamin B9 (folate)-enhanced rice [40, 41]. Conventional breeding techniques could not be applied due to the absence/low content of vitamin A in rice grain. For Golden Rice, daffodil, and Pantoea genes were used to increase pro-vitamin A levels within rice endosperm [39]. The most recent version of Golden Rice has been improved further for a 23-fold increase in carotenoids [38]. Similarly, folate-biofortified rice has been generated by overexpressing Arabidopsis genes in rice endosperm. A fourfold increase in folate concentrations in rice was accomplished using this strategy [41] and in the process, folate stability for long-term storage was improved (Blancquaert et al., 2015).

Fifteen simulation analyses confirmed the positive impact of GM biofortified crop consumption on dietary intake and nutritional outcomes in humans [42]. The vast majority of these studies also confirmed that a regular portion of the targeted biofortified crop would provide the daily micronutrient requirements. For example, the recent simulation analysis of Golden Rice in Asia [43] indicated that it could reduce the prevalence of dietary vitamin A inadequacy by up to 30% (children) and 55–60% (women) in Indonesia and the Philippines, and up to 71% (children) and 78% (women) in Bangladesh.

A randomized trial on Golden Rice performed in the United States resulted in a high bio-conversion factor of β-carotene (3.8:1), by which 100 g of uncooked Golden Rice would provide about 80–100% of the estimated average requirement and 55–70% of the recommended dietary allowance (RDA) for adult men and women [44]. Currently, Golden Rice has been approved in an increasing number of countries, including the Philippines. Golden Rice and other GM biofortified crops [16, 42] would be highly cost-effective investments to reduce target micronutrient deficiencies such as vitamin A [45].

Recently, Endo et al. [46] devised a genome editing approach to produce β-carotene rice that is fast and direct, by making use of splicing variants in the Orange (Or) gene that cause β-carotene accumulation in cauliflower. The authors genome edited the orthologue of the cauliflower or gene in rice using CRISPR/Cas9 and were able to accumulate β-carotene, without having to introduce transgenes.

9. "Golden" bananas to combat vitamin A deficiency

Bananas are the world's most important fruit crop and a major staple in many African countries. Banana grows in tropical climates, where vitamin A deficiency is most prevalent [47]. The vast number of different banana varieties and the highly variable distribution of vitamin A levels make them amenable for biofortification using biotechnology. Unfortunately, the cooking banana East African highland banana (EAHB) consumed in Uganda as a staple for tens of millions of people has low vitamin A levels.

As bananas are difficult to breed, genetic engineering of bananas with increased vitamin A content has been critical to improving vitamin A levels. The bulk of the research has been performed on the Cavendish banana, most popular in the Western Hemisphere. As a result, the Cavendish has been used as a model system for the EAHB. High levels of vitamin A (20 lg/g dry weight) were found in transgenic banana lines expressing phytoene synthase (derived from the fruit of the Fe'I banana found in Papa New Guinea, which only grows in small bunches) under the control of the banana ubiquitone promoter (Ubi). These transgenic lines appear as dark yellow-orange in color and can provide improved nutrition to some of the poorest subsistence farmers in Africa. Consumption of 300 g of transgenic banana could provide as much as 50% of vitamin A required per person per day. Although there is no existing regulatory framework for biotechnology that is currently set up in Uganda, early release is hoped for [48]. More recently, Kaur et al. [49] demonstrated the capability of genome editing to increase β-carotene accumulation in Cavendish banana. The authors created indels in the lycopene epsilon-cyclase (LCYε) gene to increase β-carotene content.

10. Biofortified maize, cassava, and sweet potato

Maize also produces β-carotene, and concentrations vary greatly between different varieties. Although β-carotene content can be increased using conventional breeding, genetic engineering strategies have also been implemented. Consumption of transgenic maize biofortified with β-carotene improved volunteer's health in clinical trials held in Africa and North America [50, 51]. Moreover, chickens fed transgenic biofortified maize produced eggs that exhibited increased carotenoid content [52]. The deep orange color of biofortified maize challenges public perception for some African populaces, as orange maize is often associated with animal feed, whereas white maize is traditionally considered to be for human consumption.

The BioCassava Plus project specifically targets cassava, a staple crop in Africa that is nutritionally deficient yet is consumed by a quarter of a million sub-Saharan Africans [53]. Transgenic cassava expressing high levels of β-carotene have been demonstrated to increase vitamin A levels and improve nutritional status in feeding studies [54]. Programs such as the BioCassava Project could therefore generate cassava crops with lasting nutritional benefits.

β-Carotene biofortified sweet potato has become a priority for sub-Saharan Africa [55]. White-fleshed sweet potato was transformed with the Orange (Or) gene responsible for carotenoid accumulation, so that β-carotene and total carotenoids levels in the IbOr-Ins transgenic sweet potato were 10-fold higher compared to that of white-fleshed sweet potato [56, 57].

11. Conclusions

This chapter illustrates the ability of biofortification using genetic engineering to address micronutrient deficiencies in a variety of crops found in resource-poor nations. The current regulatory climate and anti-GMO lobbying efforts have retarded the release of GM crops that address highly prevalent vitamin and mineral deficiencies [58, 59]. Nevertheless, the proof of concept has been realized for various nutritionally enhanced GMOs [37, 60]. This has triggered an increase in the number of nutritional traits in the global GM crops pipeline over the last two decades and is expected to be further reinforced in the near future [61]. Consumer opinion on nutritious crops is hardly affected by the type of technology used to generate them [45, 62]. It is unfortunate that a significant effect of lobbying polarizes public opinion, regardless of the scientific basis of given arguments [63]. The current environment is showing signs of turning around with the approval of Golden Rice in several countries. It is anticipated that other biofortified crops will soon follow regulatory approval, and thus help to alleviate malnutrition worldwide.

Author details

Kathleen Hefferon
Department of Microbiology, Cornell University, Ithaca, NY, USA

*Address all correspondence to: klh22@cornell.edu

References

[1] Kumar S, Palve A, Joshi C, Srivastava RK, Shekh R. Crop biofortification for iron (Fe), zinc (Zn) and vitamin A with transgenic approaches. Heliyon. 2019;**5**(6):e01914. DOI: 10.1016/j.heliyon.2019.e01914

[2] Hirschi KA. Nutrient biofortification of food crops. Annual Review of Nutrition. 2009;**29**:401-421

[3] Bhullar NK, Gruissem W. Nutritional enhancement of rice for human health: The contribution of biotechnology. Biotechnology Advances. 2013;**31**:50-57

[4] Grusak MA, DellaPenna G. Composition of plants to enhance human nutrition and health. Annual Review of Plant Physiology and Plant Molecular Biology. 1999;**50**:133-161

[5] Miret JA, Munné-Bosch S. Plant amino acid-derived vitamins: Biosynthesis and function. Amino Acids. 2014;**46**:809-824

[6] Bouis HE, Welch RM. Biofortification—A sustainable agricultural strategy for reducing micronutrient malnutrition in the global south. Crop Science. 2010;**50**:S20-S32

[7] Amarakoon D, Thavarajah D, McPhee K, Thavarajah P. Iron-, zinc-, and magnesium-rich field peas (*Pisum sativum* L.) with naturally low phytic acid: A potential food-based solution to global micronutrient malnutrition. Journal of Food Composition and Analysis. 2012;**27**:8-13

[8] Gómez-Galera S, Rojas E, Sudhakar D, Zhu C, Pelacho AM, Capell T, et al. Critical evaluation of strategies for mineral fortification of staple food crops. Transgenic Research. 2010;**19**:165-180

[9] White PJ, Broadley MR. Biofortification of crops with seven mineral elements often lacking in human diets—Iron, zinc, copper, calcium, magnesium, selenium and iodine. New Phytologist. 2009;**182**:49-84

[10] White PJ, Broadley MR. Biofortifying crops with essential mineral elements. Trends in Plant Science. 2005;**10**:586-593

[11] Fageria VD. Nutrient interactions in crop plants. Journal of Plant Nutrition. 2006;**24**:1269-1290

[12] Rossi G, Figliolia A, Socciarelli FS. Zinc and copper bioaccumulation in *Brassica napus* at flowering and maturation. Engineering in Life Sciences. 2004;**4**:271-275

[13] Briat J-F, Fobis-Loisy I, Grignon N, Lobréaux S, Pascal N, Savino G, et al. Cellular and molecular aspects of iron metabolism in plants. Biology of the Cell. 1995;**84**:69-81

[14] Brown JJ. Mechanism of iron uptake by plants. Plant, Cell & Environment. 1978;**1**:249-257

[15] Vazquez MD, Barcelo J, Poschenrieder C, Madico J, Hatton P, Baker AJM, et al. Localization of zinc and cadmium in *Thlaspi caerulescens* (Brassicaceae), a metalophyte that can hyperaccumulate both metals. Journal of Plant Physiology. 1992;**140**:350-355

[16] Vazquez MD, Poschenrieder C, Barcelo J, Baker AJM, Hatton P, Cope GH. Compartmentation of zinc in roots and leaves of the zinc hyperaccumulator *Thlaspi caerulescens* J & C Presl. Botanica Acta. 1994;**107**:243-250

[17] Morrissey J, Guerinot M-L. Iron uptake and transport in plants: The good, the bad, and the ionome. Chemical Reviews. 2009;**109**(10):4553-4567

[18] Masuda H, Aung MS, Nishizawa NK. Iron biofortification of rice using different transgenic approaches. Rice. 2013;**6**:40

[19] Li S, Liu X, Zhou X, Li Y, Yang W, Chen R. Improving zinc and iron accumulation in maize grains using the zinc and iron transporter ZmZIP5. Plant & Cell Physiology. 2019;**60**(9):2077-2085. DOI: 10.1093/pcp/pcz104

[20] Beasley JT, Bonneau JP, Sánchez-Palacios JT, Moreno-Moyano LT, Callahan DL, Tako E, et al. Metabolic engineering of bread wheat improves grain iron concentration and bioavailability. Plant Biotechnology Journal. 2019;**17**(8):1514-1526. DOI: 10.1111/pbi.13074

[21] Sharma R, Yeh KC. The dual benefit of a dominant mutation in Arabidopsis IRON DEFICIENCY TOLERANT1 for iron biofortification and heavy metal phytoremediation. Plant Biotechnology Journal. May 2020;**18**(5):1200-1210. DOI: 10.1111/pbi.13285

[22] Qiao K, Wang F, Liang S, Wang H, Hu Z, Chai T. New biofortification tool: Wheat TaCNR5 enhances zinc and manganese tolerance and increases zinc and manganese accumulation in rice grains. Journal of Agricultural and Food Chemistry. 2019;**67**(35):9877-9884. DOI: 10.1021/acs.jafc.9b04210

[23] Aung M-A, Masuda H, Kobayashi T, Nakanishi H, Yamakawa T, Nishizawa NK. Iron biofortification of Myanmar rice. Frontiers in Plant Science. 2013;**4**:158

[24] Paul S, Ali N, Datta SK, Datta K. Development of an iron-enriched high-yieldings indica rice cultivar by introgression of a high-iron trait from transgenic iron-biofortified rice. Plant Foods for Human Nutrition. 2014;**69**:203-208

[25] Trijatmiko KR, Dueñas C, Tsakirpaloglou N, Torrizo L, Arines FM, Adeva C, et al. Biofortified indica rice attains iron and zinc nutrition dietary targets in the field. Scientific Reports. 2016;**6**:19792

[26] Banakar R, Fernandez A-A, Díaz-Benito P, Abadia J, Capell T, Christou P. Phytosiderophores determine thresholds for iron and zinc accumulation in biofortified rice endosperm while inhibiting the accumulation of cadmium. Journal of Experimental Botany. 2017;**68**(17):4983-4995

[27] Tan GZH, Das Bhowmik SS, Hoang TML, Karbaschi MR, Long H, Cheng A, et al. Investigation of baseline iron levels in Australian chickpea and evaluation of a transgenic biofortification approach. Frontiers in Plant Science. 2018;**9**:788

[28] Manwaring HR, Bligh HF, Yadav R. The challenges and opportunities associated with biofortification of pearl millet (*Pennisetum glaucum*) with elevated levels of grain iron and zinc. Frontiers in Plant Science. 2016;**23**:7

[29] Narayanan N, Beyene G, Chauhan RD, Gaitán-Solis E, Grusak MA, Taylor N, et al. Overexpression of Arabidopsis VIT1 increases accumulation of iron in cassava roots and stems. Plant Science. 2015;**240**:170-181

[30] Dayod M, Tyerman SD, Leigh RA, Gilliham M. Calcium storage in plants and the implications for calcium biofortification. Protoplasma. 2010;**247**:215-231

[31] Park S, Elless MP, Park J, Jenkins A, Lim W, Chambers E, et al. Sensory analysis of calcium-biofortified lettuce. Plant Biotechnology Journal. 2009;**7**:106-117

[32] Connolly EL. Raising the bar for biofortification: Enhanced levels of

bioavailable calcium in carrots. Trends in Biotechnology. 2008;**26**:401-403

[33] Martínez-Ballesta MC, Dominguez-Perles R, Moreno DA, Muries B, Alcaraz-López C, Bastías E, et al. Minerals in plant food: Effect of agricultural practices and role in human health. A review. Agronomy and Sustainable Development. 2010;**30**:295-309

[34] Ishikawa T, Dowdle J, Smirnoff N. Progress in manipulating ascorbic acid biosynthesis and accumulation in plants. Physiologia Plantarum. 2006;**126**:343-355

[35] Smith AG, Croft MT, Moulin M, Webb ME. Plants need their vitamins too. Current Opinion in Plant Biology. 2007;**10**:266-275

[36] Beyer P. Golden rice and 'golden' crops for human nutrition. New Biotechnology. 2010;**27**:478-481

[37] de Steur H, Blancquaert D, Strobbe S, Lambert W, Gellynck X, Van Der Straeten D. Status and market potential of transgenic biofortified crops. Nature Biotechnology. 2015;**33**:25-29

[38] Paine JA, Shipton CA, Chaggar S, Howells RM, Kennedy MJ, Vernon G, et al. Improving the nutritional value of Golden Rice through increased pro-vitamin A content. Nature Biotechnology. 2005;**4**:482-487

[39] Ye X, Al-Babili S, Klöti A, Zhang J, Lucca P, Beyer P, et al. Engineering the provitamin A (β-carotene) biosynthetic pathway into (carotenoid-free) rice endosperm. Science. 2000;**287**:303-305

[40] Blancquaert D, de Steur H, Gellynck X, Van Der Straeten D. Present and future of folate biofortification of crop plants. Journal of Experimental Botany. 2014;**65**:895-906

[41] Storozhenko S, de Brouwer V, Volckaert M, Navarrete O, Blancquaert D, Zhang GF, et al. Folate fortification of rice by metabolic engineering. Nature Biotechnology. 2007;**25**:1277-1279

[42] De Steur H, Mehta S, Gellynck X, Finkelstein JL. GM biofortified crops: Potential effects on targeting the micronutrient intake gap in human populations. Current Opinion in Biotechnology. 2017a;**44**:181-188

[43] de Moura FF, Moursi M, Angel MD, Angeles-Agdeppa I, Atmarita A, Gironella GM, et al. Biofortified β-carotene rice improves vitamin A intake and reduces the prevalence of inadequacy among women and young children in a simulated analysis in Bangladesh, Indonesia, and the Philippines. The American Journal of Clinical Nutrition. 2016;**104**:769-775

[44] Tang G, Qin J, Dolnikowski GG, Russell RM, Grusak MA. Golden Rice is an effective source of vitamin A. American Journal of Clinical Nutrition. 2009;**89**:1776-1783

[45] de Steur H, Wesana J, Blancquaert D, van der Straeten D, Gellynck X. The socio-economics of genetically modified biofortified crops: A systematic review and meta-analysis. Annals of the New York Academy of Sciences. 2017c;**1390**:14-33

[46] Endo A, Saika H, Takemura M, Misawa N, Toki S. A novel approach to carotenoid accumulation in rice callus by mimicking the cauliflower Orange mutation via genome editing. Rice (N Y). 2019;**12**(1):81. DOI: 10.1186/s12284-019-0345-3

[47] Amah D, van Biljon A, Brown A, Perkins-Veazie P, Swennen R, Labuschagne M. Recent advances in banana (*Musa* spp.) biofortification to alleviate vitamin A deficiency. Critical

Reviews in Food Science and Nutrition. 2018;**12**:1-39

[48] Paul JY, Harding R, Tushemereirwe W, Dale J. Banana 21: From gene discovery to deregulated Golden bananas. Frontiers in Plant Sciences. 2018;**9**:558

[49] Kaur N, Alok A, Shivani KP, Kaur N, Awasthi P, Chaturvedi S, et al. CRISPR/Cas9 directed editing of lycopene epsilon-cyclase modulates metabolic flux for β-carotene biosynthesis in banana fruit. Metabolic Engineering. 2020;**59**:76-86. DOI: 10.1016/j.ymben.2020.01.008

[50] Li S, Nugroho A, Rocheford T, White WS. Vitamin A equivalence of the β-carotene in β-carotene-biofortified maize porridge consumed by women. American Journal of Clinical Nutrition. 2010;**92**:1105-1112

[51] Mugode L, Ha B, Kaunda A, Sikombe T, Phiri S, Mutale R, et al. Carotenoid retention of biofortified provitamin A maize (*Zea mays* L.) after Zambian traditional methods of milling, cooking and storage. Journal of Agricultural and Food Chemistry. 2014;**62**:6317-6325

[52] Moreno JA, Díaz-Gómez J, Nogareda C, Angulo E, Sandmann G, Portero-Otin M, et al. The distribution of carotenoids in hens fed on biofortified maize is influenced by feed composition, absorption, resource allocation and storage. Scientific Reports. 2016;**6**:35346

[53] Sayre R, Beeching JR, Cahoon EB, Egesi C, Fauquet C, Fellman J, et al. The BioCassava plus program: Biofortification of cassava for sub-Saharan Africa. Annual Reviews of Plant Biology. 2011;**62**:251-272

[54] Talsma EF, Brouwer ID, Verhoef H, Mbera GNK, Mwangi AM, Demir AY, et al. Biofortified yellow cassava and vitamin A status of Kenyan children: A randomized controlled trial. The American Journal of Clinical Nutrition. 2016;**103**:258-267

[55] Fuglie KO. Priorities for sweetpotato research in developing countries: Results of a survey. HortScience. 2007;**42**:1200-1206

[56] Kim SH, Ahn YO, Ahn MJ, Jeong JC, Lee HS, Kwak SS. Cloning and characterization of an orange gene that increases carotenoid accumulation and salt stress tolerance in transgenic sweetpotato cultures. Plant Physiology and Biochemistry. 2013;**70**:445-454

[57] Park SC, Kim HS, Park SU, Lee JS, Park WS, Ahn MJ, et al. Enhanced accumulation of carotenoids in sweetpotato plants overexpressing IbOr-Ins gene in purple-fleshed sweetpotato cultivar. Plant Physiology and Biochemistry. 2015;**86**:82-90

[58] Moghissi AA, Pei S, Liu Y. Golden rice: Scientific, regulatory and public information processes of a genetically modified organism. Critical Reviews in Biotechnology. 2016;**36**:535-541

[59] Potrykus I. The GMO-crop potential for more, and more nutritious food is blocked by unjustified regulation. Journal of Innovation & Knowledge. 2017;**2**:90-96

[60] van der Straeten D, Fitzpatrick TB, de Steur H. Editorial overview: Biofortification of crops: Achievements, future challenges, socio-economic, health and ethical aspects. Current Opinion in Biotechnology. 2017;**44**:7-10

[61] Parisi C, Tillie P, Rodríguez-Cerezo E. The global pipeline of GM crops out to 2020. Nature Biotechnology. 2016;**34**:31

[62] De Steur H, Wesana J, Blancquaert D, van der Straeten D, Gellynck X. Methods matter: A meta-regression on the determinants of willingness-to-pay studies on biofortified foods. Annals of the New York Academy of Sciences. 2017b;**1390**:34-46

[63] Wesseler J, Zilberman D. The economic power of the Golden Rice opposition. Environment and Development Economics. 2014;**19**:724-742

Chapter 3

Vitamins

Mohanad Mousa Kareem and Majid S. Jabir

Abstract

This chapter is going to explain a part of the nutrients the human body needs. They are organic compounds called vitamins. Those compounds will be clarified, as well as their benefits, deficiencies, chemical structure, and why the body needs them crucially. Vitamins is an exceptionally vital recognized name required in certain amounts in the body, some of them exist as a complicated natural compounds found in herbal meals. It plays a key function in regular metabolism, the absence of which in the diet causes deficiency and several diseases. Vitamins are differentiated from the trace elements, also found in the weight-reduction plan in small quantities for health, growth, replica, and other crucial metabolism.

Keywords: vitamins, water-soluble vitamins, fat-soluble vitamins, deficiency, benefits, dosage

1. Introduction

The human body is a magnificent machine, and to function well, the body needs certain supplements. Vitamins are one of the most essential elements for the body. There are nutrients that the body can make on its own, and there are others that the body is not able to make. Vitamins are one of the nutrients that the body is unable to make, so they must be consumed from aliments. Vitamins are an organic molecule, which is an essential micronutrient that an organism needs for its metabolism to function. They are divided into two groups, fat-soluble vitamins and water-soluble vitamins. The first group contains vitamins A, D, E, and K, while the second consists of thiamin (B1), riboflavin (B2), niacin (B3), pantothenic acid (B5), pyridoxal, pyridoxamine, pyridoxine (B6), biotin-cobalamin (B12), folic acid, and ascorbic acid [1–10].

2. Fat-soluble vitamins

They are a type that is absorbed well into the blood stream via fatty nourishments and are stored in limited amounts; they can be easy to separate and disposed out from the body through urine [8–10].

2.1 Vitamin A

Vitamin A is a yellow viscous liquid alicyclic alcohol $C_{20}H_{30}O$ that contains one more double bond in a molecule than vitamin A1 and is less active biologically in mammals and that occurs especially in the liver oil of freshwater fish. It consists of three biologically active molecules, retinol, retinal (retinaldehyde), and retinoic acid, all derived from the plant precursor molecule, β-carotene (**Figure 1**) [11, 12].

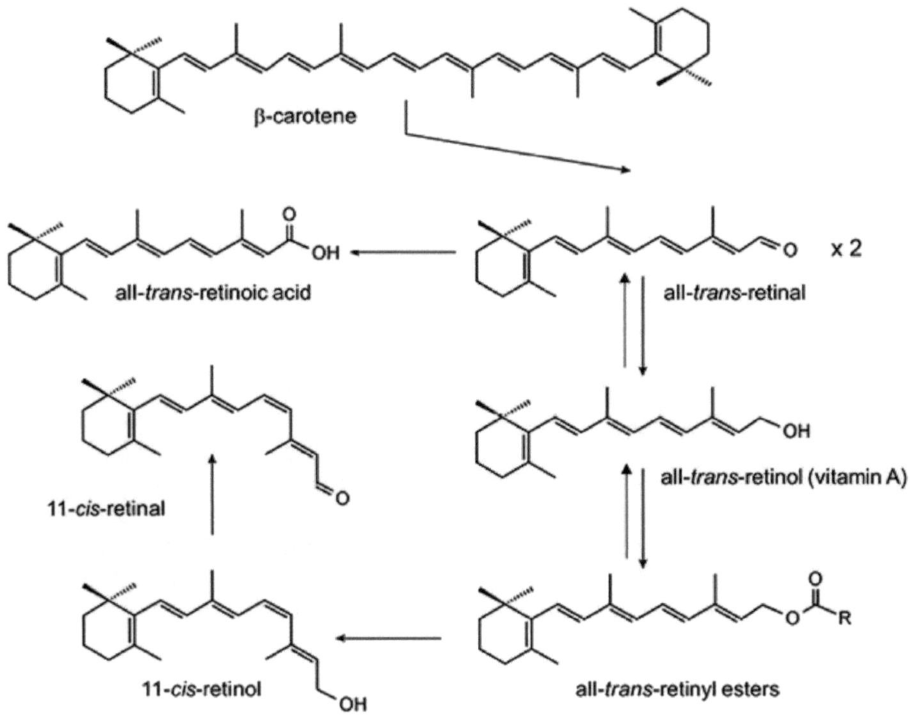

Figure 1.
Types of vitamin A.

Retinol also functions in the synthesis of certain glycoproteins and mucopolysaccharides necessary for mucous production and normal growth regulation. Retinol is the predominant, active form of vitamin A found in the blood. Retinyl palmitate is the storage form of the vitamin [13].

This vitamin is important to the body for playing an effective role in growth and development, the visual system, immunity, and reproduction as well as supplying epithelial cellular integrity. Most of the vitamin A is stored in the liver in the form of retinyl esters. Sources of vitamin A vary from vegetables to fruits and are found in animal-sourced foods, such as eggs, oily fish, liver, cheese, and butter. The lack of this vitamin can leave severe effects on the function of the body such as night blindness, decreased resistance to infections, and extremely dry skin, hair, or nails. Just deficiency can be harmful; the overuse of vitamin A can be toxic and lead to hypervitaminosis. An average dose of this vitamin needed for the body is 0.7 mg for men and 0.6 mg for women on a daily diet. Women who have been through menopause and older men, who are more at risk of osteoporosis, should avoid having more than 1.5 mg of vitamin A per day from food and supplements [7, 13, 14].

2.2 Vitamin D

Vitamin D is a steroid vitamin, which promotes the intestinal absorption and metabolism of calcium and phosphorus. There are two main types of vitamin D, Vitamin D_2, which is synthesized by plants and is not created by the human body. Vitamin D_3, which is made in large amounts in the skin when daylight strikes uncovered skin. Moreover, it can be ingested from animal sources. As well as there other types like ergosterol, dehydrocholesterol, and the biologically active form of the hormone 1,25-dihydroxy vitamin D_3 termed calcitriol.

Vitamin D is not active itself (it is a prohormone); it is modified to yield biologically active forms, such as calcitriol. Calcitriol (derived from vitamin D) is a transcription factor, influencing expression of proteins involved in calcium absorption and transport [15–17] (**Figure 2**).

Vitamin D is required to maintain normal blood levels of calcium and phosphate, which in turn is needed for the normal mineralization of the bone, muscle contraction, nerve conduction, general cellular function in all cells of the body and supporting lung function, and cardiovascular health. It may also protect against a range of diseases and conditions, such as type 1 diabetes. Vitamin D also modulates the transcription of cell cycle proteins, which decrease cell proliferation and increase cell differentiation of a number of specialized cells of the body (e.g., osteoclastic precursors, enterocytes, and keratinocytes). This property may explain the actions of vitamin D in bone resorption, intestinal calcium transport, and skin. Vitamin D also possesses immunomodulatory properties that may alter responses to infections in vivo. These cell-differentiating and immunomodulatory properties underlie the reason why vitamin D derivatives now are in use successfully in the treatment of psoriasis and other skin disorders. Oily fish, such as salmon, sardines, herring, and mackerel, contain a fair amount of vitamin D as well as red meat, liver, egg yolks, and fortified foods, such as most fat spreads and some breakfast cereals. Another source of vitamin D is dietary supplements [15–18].

The simplest way to get all the vitamin D the body needs is from direct sunlight. The absence of this very vitamin in an adult daily diet can result in hypovitaminosis

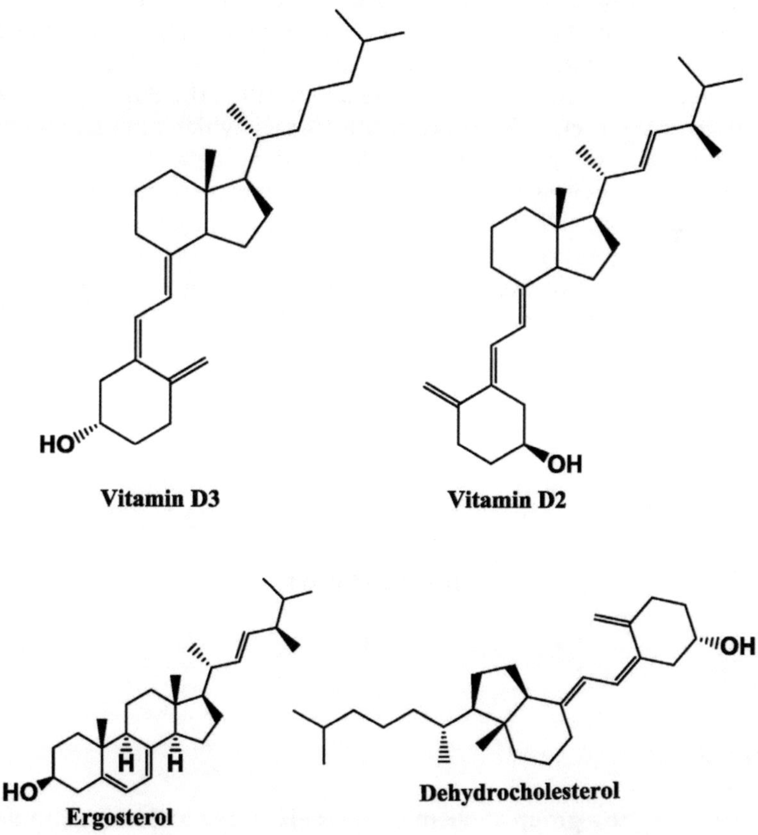

Figure 2.
Types of vitamin D.

D, which leads to loss of bone density, which can contribute to osteoporosis and fractures (broken bones). In children, a severe vitamin D deficiency can cause delays in growth as well as rickets, a disease where the bones become soft and bend. Furthermore, vitamin D deficiency has been in link with several cancers, type 1 diabetes, multiple sclerosis, high blood pressure, and thyroid problems. A daily dose of vitamin D 1000 IU should prevent very low vitamin D levels and should be sufficient to help most aging adults get the benefit [17–19].

2.3 Vitamin E

Vitamin E is a major lipid-soluble antioxidant in the cell's antioxidant defense system and is exclusively obtained from the diet. The term "vitamin E" refers to a family of eight naturally occurring homologs synthesized by plants from homogentisic acid. All are derivatives of 6-chromanol and differ in the number and position of methyl groups on the ring structure known as tocopherols (**Figure 3**) [20].

This particular vitamin plays a huge role in protecting cell membranes and other fat-soluble parts of the body (LDL cholesterol) from oxidation; it also may reduce the risk of heart disease, discourage development of some types of cancer, promote normal growth and development, and promote normal red blood cell formation. It can also act as an anti-blood clotting agent and plays some role in the body's ability to process glucose. In addition, it is recognized to aid the process of wound healing. This vitamin is found in wheat germ oil, vegetable oils, nuts and seeds, whole grains, and egg yolk, in addition to leafy green vegetables [21, 22].

Vitamin E is mainly stored in the liver before released into the blood stream for use. Vitamin E is essential to the central nervous system. It is among the body's main antioxidants, and a deficiency results in oxidative stress, which can lead to muscle weakness. A deficiency can cause certain neurons, called the Purkinje neurons, to break down, harming their ability to transmit signals, which causes walking difficulties. Numbing and tingling also is a sign of deficiency, and the damage to nerve fibers can prevent the nerves from transmitting signals correctly, resulting in these sensations, which is also called peripheral neuropathy. The deficiency can also cause weakness of light receptors in the retina and other cells in the eye, and this can lead to loss of vision over time as well as immune system problems. The recommended daily dosage of this vitamin for males is 30 IU and for females 24 IU [22–24].

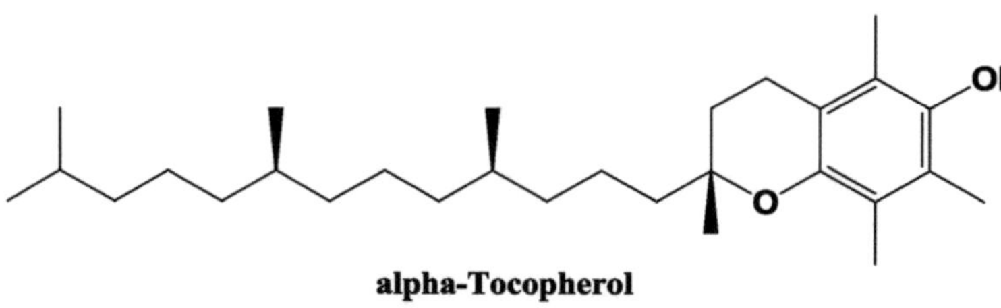

Figure 3.
Vitamin E.

2.4 Vitamin K

Vitamin K refers to a group of chemically similar fat-soluble compounds called naphthoquinones: vitamin K1 (phytonadione) is found in plants and is the primary source of vitamin K for humans through dietary consumption, vitamin K2 compounds (menaquinones) are made by bacteria in the human gut, and vitamin K3 (menadione) is a water-soluble preparation available for adults only (**Figure 4**).

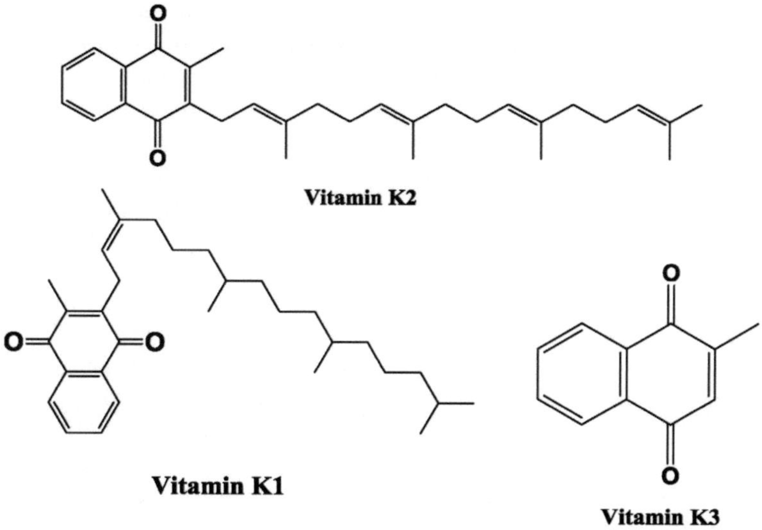

Figure 4.
Types of vitamin K.

Vitamin K is necessary for the liver to produce the coagulation factors II, VII, IX, and X as well as the clotting factors protein C, protein S, and protein Z [25, 26].

The body needs vitamin K to produce prothrombin, a protein and clotting factor that is important in blood clotting and bone metabolism. Vitamin K1, or phylloquinone, comes from plants. It is the main type of dietary vitamin K. A lesser source is vitamin K2, or menaquinones, which occurs in some animal-based and fermented foods. The body is in need for both types of vitamin K to produce prothrombin, a protein that plays crucial roles in blood clotting, bone metabolism, and heart health. Vitamin K also helps facilitate energy production in the mitochondria of cells. Vitamin K has antioxidant properties. It protects cellular membranes from damage due to excess free radicals, in a process known as peroxidation. It is in use in synthesizing gamma-carboxyglutamate, a posttranslationally modified amino acid in prothrombin. Green vegetables contain the highest amounts of vitamin K like kale, spinach, turnip greens, collards, and green leaf lettuce vegetables, but there are many other good sources like fish, liver, meat, eggs, and cereals (contain smaller amounts). Vitamin K is made as well by the bacteria in the lower intestinal tract. Vitamin K deficiency is very rare. It occurs when the body does not properly absorb the vitamin from the intestinal tract. Vitamin K deficiency can also occur after long-term treatment with antibiotics. In adults, primary vitamin K-deficient states that manifest as bleeding are almost unknown, except when the absorption of the vitamin is impaired, resulting in an underlying pathology. Vitamin K deficiency bleeding is a problem that occurs in some newborns. It happens during the first few days of life. This condition used to be named hemorrhagic disease of the newborn. About toxicity, natural vitamin K seems free of toxic side effects. This apparent safety is designated out by the common clinical administration of phylloquinone at doses of 10–20 mg or greater. The recommended daily dosage for male adults is 120 mcg and for female adults is 90 mcg [26–29].

3. Water-soluble vitamins

3.1 Thiamin (B1)

Thiamin is one of the B vitamins. The B vitamins are a group of water-soluble vitamins that are part of many of the chemical reactions in the body. It plays a role by producing energy from carbohydrates and helping in proper nerve function as well as stabilizing the appetite and promoting growth and good muscle tone. It is also involved in the flow of electrolytes into and out of muscle and nerve cells. Thiamin is rapidly converted to its active form, thiamin pyrophosphate (TPP) (**Figure 5**), in the brain and liver by specific enzymes, thiamine phosphotransferase [30, 31].

There are many natural ways to add thiamine-rich foods to an everyday diet. Food sources of thiamine include beef, liver, dried milk, nuts, oats, oranges, pork, eggs, seeds, legumes, peas, and yeast. Foods also are fortified with thiamine. Some foods that are fortified with B1 are rice, pasta, breads, cereals, and flour. The relieving thing about thiamin is that it's non-toxic even at high dosage. However, the deficiency can be worrying because it leads to loss of appetite, weakness, and tiredness. Also causes insomnia, loss of weight, in addition to depression and gastrointestinal problems. Moreover, the deficiency leads to neurological problems and beriberi, which is a muscle atrophy. Furthermore, we must mention Wernicke-Korsakoff syndrome, which is a disease most commonly found in chronic alcoholics due to their poor dietetic lifestyles. A recommended daily dosage of thiamin for body requirement is 1.0–1.5 mg for normal adults [32–34].

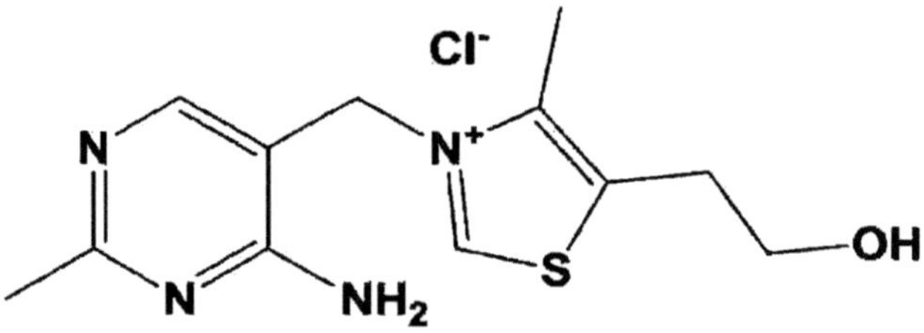

Thiamin

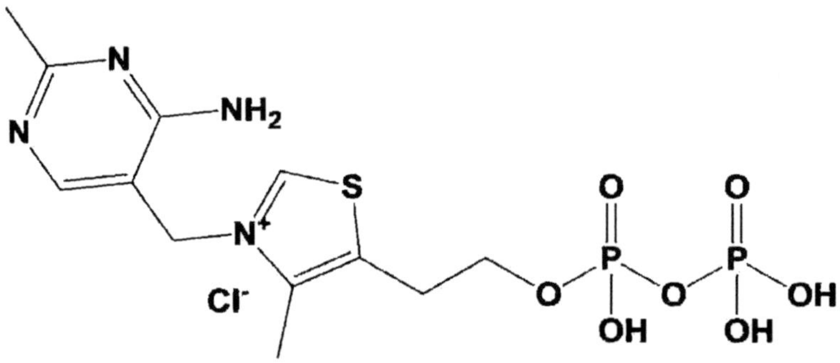

Thiamin Pyrophosphate

Figure 5.
Types of vitamin B1.

3.2 Riboflavin (B2)

Vitamin B2 is an organic compound that is not stored by the body except in insignificant amounts. It must be replenished daily. It is the precursor of coenzymes flavin mononucleotide (FMN) and flavin adenine dinucleotide (FAD) (**Figure 6**). The enzymes that require FMN or FAD and $FADH_2$ as cofactors are termed flavoproteins. Several flavoproteins also contain metal ions, termed metalloflavoproteins. It contributes in energy production carbohydrate, fat, and protein metabolism and also in the formation of antibodies and red blood cells, not to mention respiration and maintenance of good vision and alleviating skin, nails, and hair, plus improving eye fatigue [35–37].

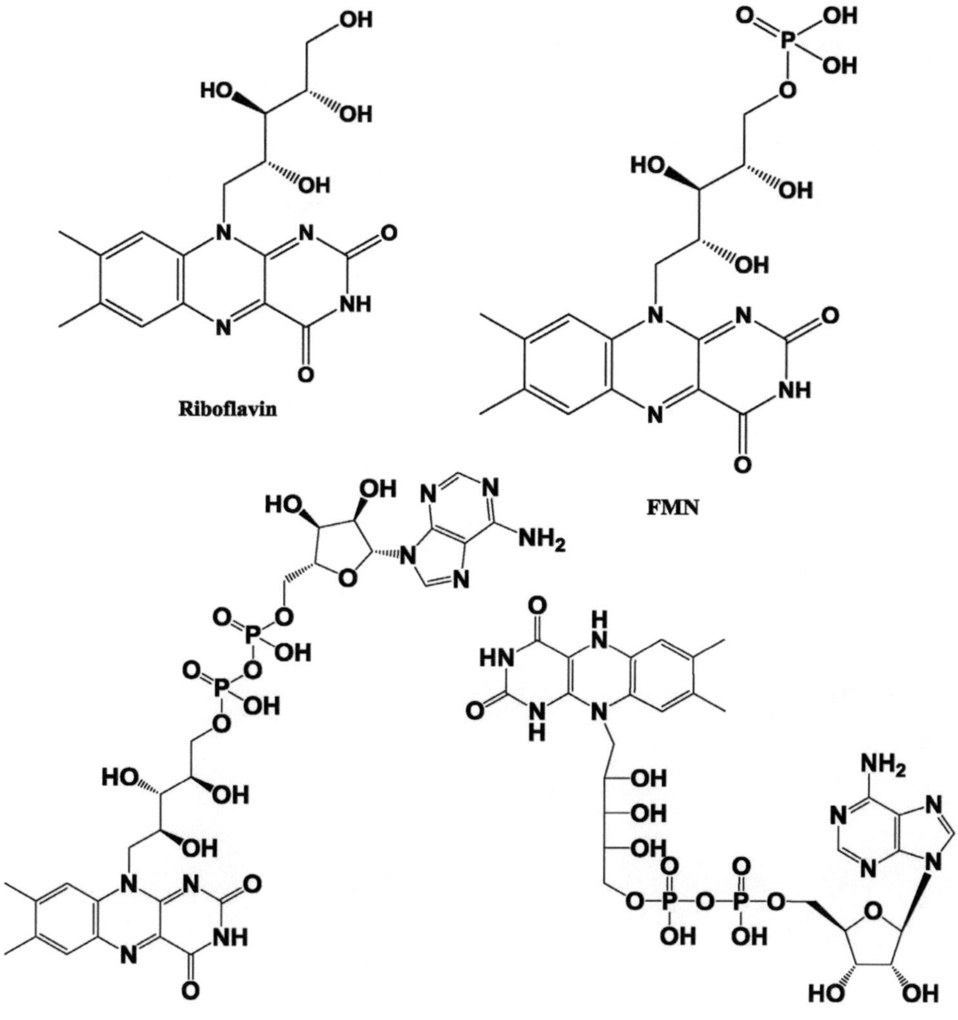

Riboflavin

FMN

FAD

FADH2

Figure 6.
Types of vitamin B2.

Riboflavin decomposes when exposed to visible light. This characteristic can lead to riboflavin deficiencies in newborns treated for hyperbilirubinemia by phototherapy. Sources of riboflavin are present in large amounts in meat, fish, eggs, vegetables, dairy foods, and grain products. The deficiency of B2 is common due to poor diet. The resulting side effects of the deficiency of riboflavin are itching, burning eyes, cracks and sores in mouth and lips. In addition to bloodshot eyes, dermatitis, oily skin, and digestive disturbances. Moreover, normocytic anemia is associated with pure red cytoplasia of the bone marrow. The toxicity of this vitamin is not an issue due to limited intestinal absorption. The required daily dosage of B2 for adolescent and adults is 1.0–1.3 mg [10, 37, 38].

3.3 Niacin (B3)

Niacin (nicotinic acid and nicotinamide), or known as vitamin B3, is required for the synthesis of the active forms of vitamin B3, nicotinamide adenine dinucleotide (NAD+), and nicotinamide adenine dinucleotide phosphate (NADP+).

Both NAD+ and NADP+, also known as NADPH (reduced form), function as cofactors for numerous dehydrogenases (**Figure 7**) [38, 39].

Niacin is an essential nutrient required for normal metabolism, energy production, maintenance of skin and tongue, and also improvement of circulation and maintenance of nervous system as well as the health of the digestive tract. This vitamin is divided into two types, nicotinic acid and niacinamide (nicotinamide) (**Figure 8**). It helps build proteins in the skin and lock in moisture to prevent environmental damage. The use is frequent in cosmetics and personal care products due to its wonderful effectiveness and treatments to skin and hair flaws and problems. It is important to mention that niacin is highly toxic in large doses and can lead to no good; doses of only 50–100 mg nicotinic acid can cause dilation of blood vessels and potentially painful tingling ("niacin flush"), diarrhea, nausea, vomiting, and long-term liver damage. In spite of the danger, nicotonic acid regulates the cholesterol with the assistance of inositol hexaniacinate, which is a supplement that regulates cholesterol without high toxicity. Nicotinamide is nearly always safe to take, although a few cases of liver damage have been in report due to doses of over 1000 mg/day [10, 39].

This vitamin is consumed through meat like liver, fish, and pork and peanuts, whole wheat, brown rice, mushrooms, and vegetables like green peas and potatoes, as well as fruits that are enriched in B3 like avocado. Deficiency can lead to pellagra, which is a dangerous disease. The symptoms are marked by dementia,

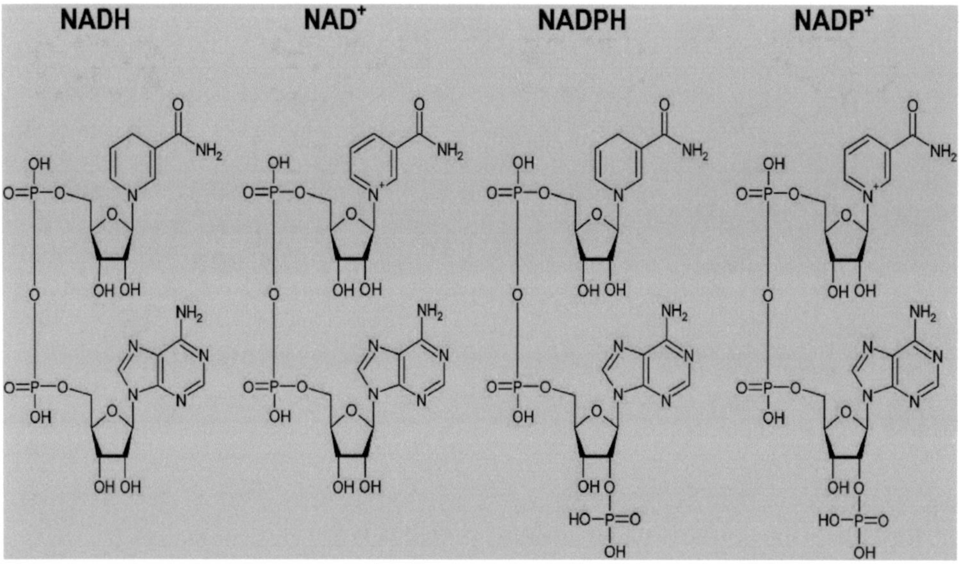

Figure 7.
Structures of NADH, NAD$^+$*, NADPH, and NADP*$^+$*.*

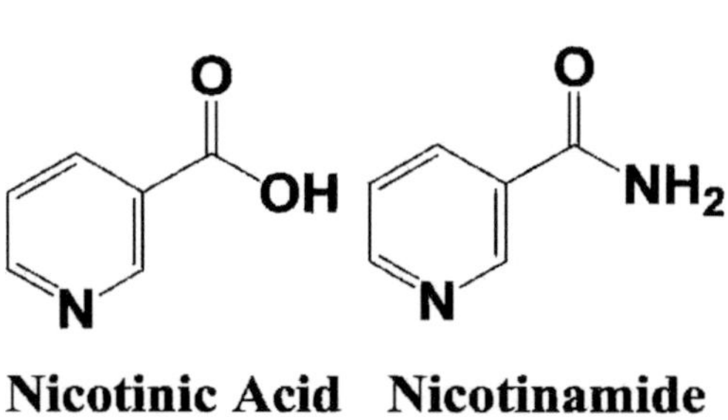

Figure 8.
Types of B3.

diarrhea, and dermatitis, also known as "the three Ds." If left untreated, pellagra can be fatal. Besides pellagra, deficiency causes gastrointestinal disturbance, loss of appetite, headache, insomnia, and mental depression. Moreover, it can be the reason of fatigue, aches, pains, nervousness, and irritability. The recommended daily dosage of a stable diet for vitamin B3 is 16 mg/day for males +14 years and for females +14 years 14 mg/day [39–41].

3.4 Pantothenic acid (B5)

Pantothenic acid (**Figure 9**) is vitamin B5. The word pantothenic comes from the Greek "pantou," meaning everywhere. Nearly all foods contain small quantities of pantothenic acid. It is one of the eight water-soluble B vitamins, which enables the body to break down carbohydrates into glucose to produce energy and to make red blood cells. This acid is formed from ß-alanine and pantoic acid. Pantothenic acid is required for the synthesis of coenzyme A (CoA) and component of the acyl carrier protein (ACP) domain of fatty acid synthase, in addition to its need for the metabolism of carbohydrate by the TCA cycle and all fats and proteins [38, 42].

Moreover, vitamin B5 also takes action in converting food into glucose, synthesizing cholesterol and forming sex and stress-related hormones in the adrenal glands. In addition, vitamin B5 helps maintain healthy skin, hair, eyes, and digestive system and also assists the body in using other vitamins. Furthermore, it can be in use for skin care as some studies have shown that vitamin B5 works as a moisturizer on the skin and enhances the healing process of skin wounds and acne. In addition, some studies suggest that vitamin B5 intake can help lower cholesterol and levels of blood triglycerides or fats. Almost all plant- and animal-based foods contain pantothenic acid in varying amounts, though food processing can cause a significant loss. Vitamin B5 is mainly found in members of the cabbage family, poultry, white and sweet potatoes, whole-grain cereals, and yeast, in addition to milk, lentils, and legumes. Deficiency is rare but can cause symptoms like headache, fatigue, irritability, impaired muscle coordination, gastrointestinal problems, and paresthesia, which is a tingling and numbing feeling in the feet, hands, legs, and other parts of the body. The recommended daily intake for this acid is 1.7–5.0 mg; large doses of pantothenic acid do not cause symptoms, other than possible diarrhea [43, 44].

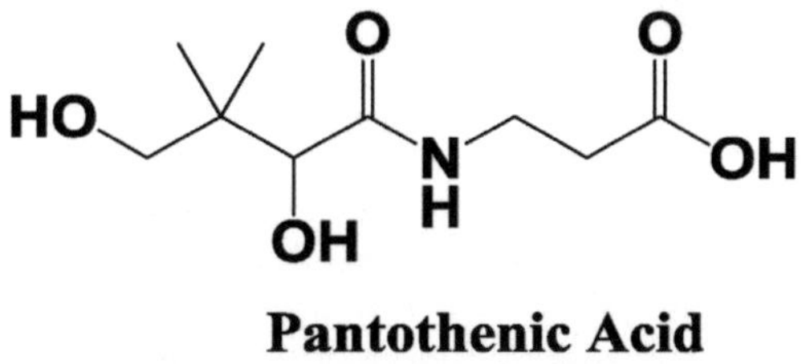

Figure 9.
Vitamin B5.

3.5 Pyridoxal, pyridoxamine, and pyridoxine (B6)

Pyridoxine is one of the vitamin B6 groups which also includes pyridoxal and pyridoxamine; all three compounds are efficiently converted by pyridoxal kinase to the biologically active form of vitamin B6, which is pyridoxal phosphate (**Figure 10**). Pyridoxal phosphate functions as a coenzyme, a substance that enhances the action of an enzyme and thereby helps catalyze and speed a biochemical reaction [38, 45].

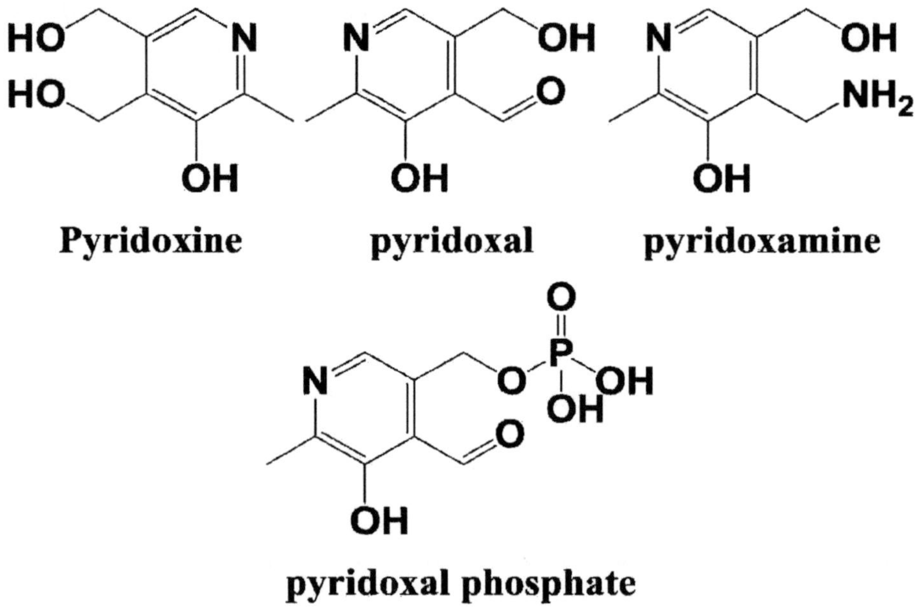

Figure 10.
Types of vitamin B6.

Vitamin B6 is important to the body for it plays a huge role in the production of red blood cells, the conversion of tryptophan to niacin (B3), and the immunity and nervous system functions. Moreover, it reduces muscle spasms, cramps, and numbness as well as maintains a proper balance of sodium and phosphorus in the body. Good sources of this vitamin is just like most other vitamins, it can be found in whole-grain cereals, eggs, vegetables, soya beans, peanuts, milk, and potatoes as well as meat like poultry, pork, and fish. The risks of the deficiency are rare but can lead to nervousness, insomnia, loss of muscle control, muscle weakness, and arm and leg cramps, in addition to water retention and skin lesions. The recommended daily dosage of this vitamin is 1.4 mg a day for men and 1.2 mg a day for women [38, 45, 46].

3.6 Biotin-cobalamin (B12)

Biotin is a water-soluble B-complex vitamin that helps the body metabolize proteins and process glucose. Biotin is also known as vitamin B7 or vitamin H (**Figure 11**). It is also involved in the metabolism of fatty acids, a type of molecule found in fats and oils and leucine, an essential amino acid that humans cannot synthesize [46].

Biotin has a number of benefits to the human body like lowering cholesterol, regulating blood sugar, improving the skin health, as well as strengthening hair and

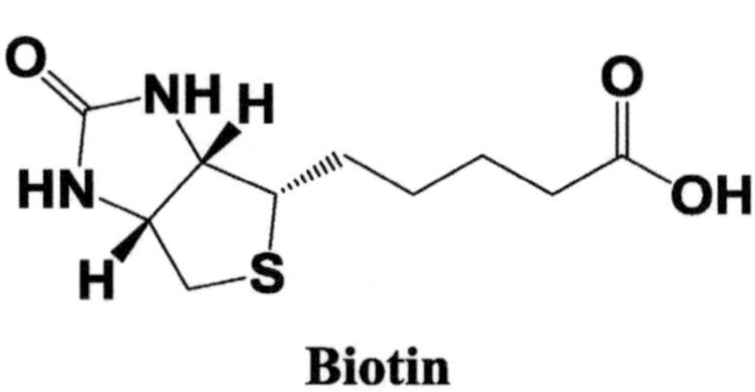

Figure 11.
Vitamin B12 (biotin).

nails. A research has found that biotin can treat multiple sclerosis, a serious disease that affects the central nervous system, if taken in high doses as studies have shown. Biotin is largely found in egg yolks, cheese, legumes such as soybeans and peanuts, leafy greens, and cauliflower. Moreover, it also exists in mushrooms, nuts and nut butters, as well as animal liver and kidney. Biotinidase deficiency (BTD) is the most common cause of biotin deficiency. BTD is a rare inherited disorder where the body is not able to use biotin and leads to biotin deficiency, which developed by a mutation in the BTD gene. This gene instructs the body on how to make the enzyme biotinidase, which the body needs to extract biotin from food. Biotin deficiency includes thinning hair, progressing to loss of hair across the body, and a scaly, red rash around body openings, including the eyes, nose, mouth, and anus, as well as development of conjunctivitis. The daily requirement of this vitamin is within 5–30 mcg, for both men and women; the dosage differs according to age [47, 48].

Cobalamin is an essential nutrient and natural water-soluble vitamin of the B-complex family that must combine with an intrinsic factor for absorption by the intestine; vitamin B12 (cyanocobalamin) (**Figure 12**) is necessary for

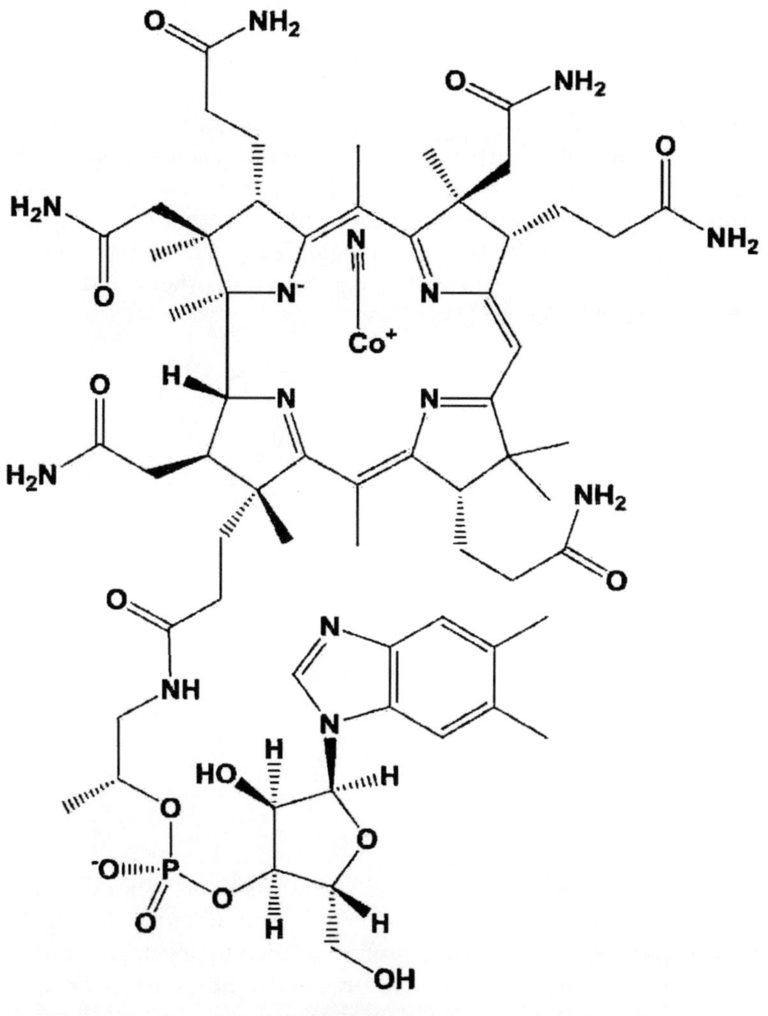

Figure 12.
Vitamin B12 (cobalamin).

hematopoiesis, which is the process by which blood cells are formed and neural, in addition to metabolism, DNA and RNA production, as well as carbohydrate, fat, and protein metabolism. B12 improves iron functions in the metabolic cycle and assists folic acid in choline synthesis. B12 metabolism is interconnected with that of folic acid. This vitamin is mainly found in meat, for instance, fish, clams, beef, animal liver and kidney, as well as in eggs, dairies, and fortified nutritional yeast. Deficiency of cobalamin results to anemia, nerve damage, and hypersensitive skin. The recommended daily requirement of this vitamin for men and women of +14 of age is 2–3 mcg/day [47–49].

3.7 Folic acid (B9)

Folic acid is a form of vitamin B9 that can dissolve in water. It is a key ingredient in the making of the nucleic acid, which forms part of all genetic material. Its main functions are synthesis and repair of DNA and RNA, aiding rapid cell division and growth, enhancing brain health, and age-related hearing loss (**Figure 13**) [50].

Folic acid is essential to the body, and the deficiency of it can cause anemia, diseases of the heart and blood vessels and defects in the brain and spinal cord in a fetus. Folic acid is added to be in study with vitamin B12 in the prevention and treatment of cancer. It is also called folate. In addition, it is in consideration that folic acid plays a preventive role in a number of conditions like autism; a recent study connected folic acid deficiency with autism. It is fair to mention that folic acid is often used to support a methotrexate prescription for rheumatoid arthritis, which is a long-term, progressive, and disabling autoimmune disease. It causes inflammation, swelling, and pain in and around the joints and other body organs. This vitamin can be consumed through legumes, eggs, leafy greens, asparagus, beetroot, citrus fruits, beef liver, wheat germ-fortified grains, and others. The required daily dosage for the body is 0.1–0.4 mg [51, 52].

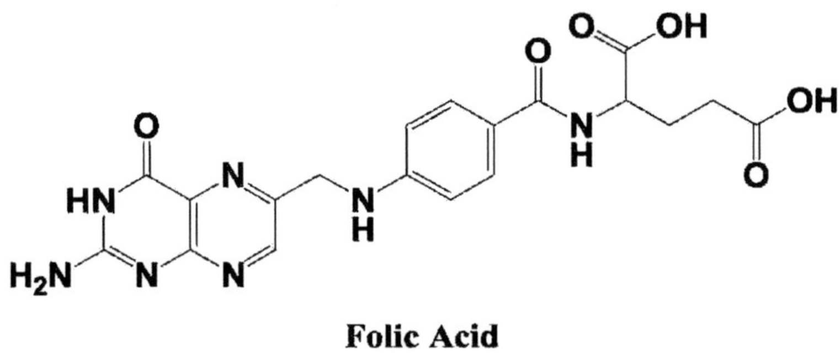

Figure 13.
Vitamin B9.

3.8 Ascorbic acid (vitamin C)

Vitamin C is also known as ascorbic acid, a water-soluble vitamin, one that is not able to be in storage by the body except in insignificant amounts. It must be replenished daily. It helps produce collagen, a protein needed to develop and maintain healthy teeth, bones, gums, cartilage, vertebrae discs, joint linings, skin, and blood vessels. Vitamin C is a powerful antioxidant that protects your cells from damage by free radicals produced by cigarette smoke, air pollution, excessive sunlight, and normal metabolism (**Figure 14**). Free radicals are considered to play a role in rapid aging and diseases such as cancer and heart disease [53–55].

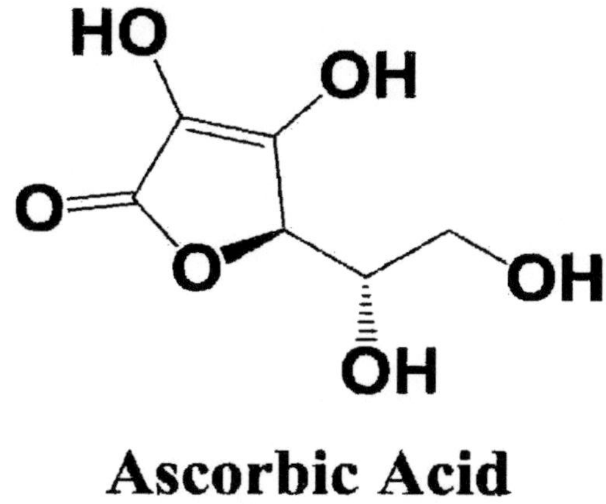

Figure 14.
Vitamin C.

It known that vitamin C helps metabolize proteins and its antioxidant activity may have a chance of reducing the risk of some cancers. Scurvy is the name for a vitamin C deficiency which results in anemia, fatigue, depression, and connective tissue defects like internal bleeding, petechiae, impaired wound healing, and gingivitis. Vitamin C is mainly found in citrus fruits such as orange, kiwi, lemon, guava, and grapefruit, and vegetables such as broccoli, cauliflower, Brussels sprouts, and capsicums are rich, natural sources of vitamin C. Other vitamin C-rich fruits include papaya, cantaloupe, and strawberries. The required intake of the vitamin is 45–60 mg for male and female, and the dosage differs according to age [54–58].

4. Conclusions

In conclusion, there are two types of vitamins, which are essential to the body, water-soluble vitamins and fat-soluble vitamins; both types play an effective part in the human body. Nobody can deny the necessity of these vitamins to the body in all ages, and the lack of it can result in severe damage in certain parts of the body according to which vitamin and age as well as the health status of each person.

Author details

Mohanad Mousa Kareem[1*] and Majid S. Jabir[2]

1 Department of Chemistry, College of Science, University of Babylon, Iraq

2 Division of Biotechnology, Department of Applied Science, University of Technology, Baghdad, Iraq

*Address all correspondence to: sci.mohanad.mousa@uobabylon.edu.iq

References

[1] Bender DA. Nutritional Biochemistry of the Vitamins. Cambridge, UK: Cambridge University Press; 2003. ISBN: 978-0-521-80388-5

[2] Herbert V, Barrett S. Vitamins and "Health" Foods: The Great American Hustle. Philadelphia: George F. Stickley Co.; 1981

[3] FDA. Consumer: Nutrition Group Warns on Vitamin Overuse. U.S. Department of Health, Education, and Welfare, Public Health Service, Food and Drug Administration; 1978;**12**:3

[4] Larrick GP. The vitamin healers. The Reporter. 1965:18-25. (quoted by R. L. Smith)

[5] Wald G. In: Sebren WH, Harris RS, editors. The Vitamins. Vol. I. New York: Academic Press; 1954

[6] Food and Nutrition Board. Dietary Reference Intakes: Applications in Dietary Assessment. Washington, DC: National Academy Press; 2001

[7] Food and Nutrition Board. Dietary Reference Intakes for Vitamin A, Vitamin K, Arsenic, Boron, Chromium, Copper, Iodine, Iron, Manganese, Molybdenum, Nickel, Silicon, Vanadium, and Zinc. Washington, DC: National Academy Press; 2002

[8] WHO/FAO. Preparation and Use of Food-Based Dietary Guidelines. Report of a Joint FAO/WHO Consultation, Nicosia, Cyprus 1996. Nutrition Program. WHO/NUT/96.6. Geneva: World Health Organization; 1996

[9] McCormick DB. Vitamin, structure and function of. In: Meyers RA, editor. Encyclopedia of Molecular Biology and Molecular Medicine. Vol. 6. Weinheim: VCH; 1997. pp. 244-252

[10] McCormick DB, Greene HL. Vitamins. In: Burtis VA, Ashwood ER, editors. Tietz Textbook of Clinical Chemistry. 2nd ed. Philadelphia: W.B. Saunders; 1994. pp. 1275-1316

[11] FAO/WHO. Requirements of vitamin A, iron, folate and vitamin B12. In: Report of a Joint FAO/WHO Expert Consultation. Food and Nutrition Series, No. 23. Rome: FAO; 1988

[12] Olson JA. Needs and sources of carotenoids and vitamin A. Nutrition Reviews. 1994;**52**(2II):S67-S73

[13] Ong DE. Absorption of vitamin A. In: Blomhoff R, editor. Vitamin A in Health and Disease. New York, NY: Marcel Dekker; 1994. pp. 37-72

[14] Stephensen CB et al. Vitamin A is excreted in the urine during acute infection. American Journal of Clinical Nutrition. 1994;**60**:388-392

[15] DeLuca HF. The vitamin D story: A collaborative effort of basic science and clinical medicine. FASEB Journal. 1988;**2**:224-236

[16] Feldman D, Glorieux FH, Pike JW. Vitamin D. New York, NY: Academic Press; 1997

[17] Pike JW. Vitamin D3 receptors: Structure and function in transcription. Annual Review of Nutrition. 1991;**11**:189-216

[18] Mawer EB, Davies M. Vitamin D deficiency, rickets and osteomalacia, a returning problem worldwide. In: Norman AW, Bouillon R, Thomasset M, editors. Vitamin D. Chemistry, Biology and Clinical Applications of the Steroid Hormone. Riverside, CA: University of California; 1997. pp. 899-906

[19] Institute of Medicine, Food and Nutrition Board. Dietary Reference Intakes for Calcium and Vitamin D. Washington, DC: National Academy Press; 2010

[20] Traber MG. Vitamin E. In: Shils ME, Shike M, Ross AC, Caballero B, Cousins R, editors. Modern Nutrition in Health and Disease. 10th ed. Baltimore, MD: Lippincott Williams & Wilkins; 2006. pp. 396-411

[21] Sen CK, Khanna S, Roy S. Tocotrienols: Vitamin E beyond tocopherols. Life Sciences. 2006;**78**:2088-2098

[22] Institute of Medicine, Food and Nutrition Board. Dietary Reference Intakes: Vitamin C, Vitamin E, Selenium, and Carotenoids. Washington, DC: National Academy Press; 2000

[23] Hathcock JN, Azzi A, Blumberg J, Bray T, Dickinson A, Frei B, et al. Vitamins E and C are safe across a broad range of intakes. The American Journal of Clinical Nutrition. 2005;**81**:736-745

[24] Horwitt MK. Interpretation of human requirements for vitamin E. In: Machlin L, editor. Vitamin E, A Comprehensive Treatise. New York, NY: Marcel Dekker; 1980. pp. 621-636

[25] Ferland G. Vitamin K. In: Erdman JW, Macdonald IA, Zeisel SH, editors. Present Knowledge in Nutrition. 10th ed. Washington, DC: Wiley-Blackwell; 2012. pp. 230-247

[26] Shearer MJ. Fat-soluble vitamins: Vitamin K. Lancet. 1995;**345**:229-234

[27] U.S. Department of Agriculture USDHHS. Dietary Guidelines for Americans. Washington, DC: U.S. Government Printing Office; 2010

[28] Booth SL, Pennington JAT, Sadowski JA. Food sources and dietary intakes of vitamin K-1 (phylloquinone) in the American diet: Data from the FDA total diet study. Journal of the American Dietetic Association. 1996;**96**:149-154

[29] Conly JM, Stein K. Quantitative and qualitative measurements of K vitamins in human intestinal contents. The American Journal of Gastroenterology. 1992;**87**:311-316

[30] Said HM. Thiamin. In: Coates PM, Betz JM, Blackman MR, et al., editors. Encyclopedia of Dietary Supplements. 2nd ed. Informa Healthcare: London and New York; 2010. pp. 748-753

[31] Bemeur C, Butterworth RF. Thiamin. In: Ross AC, Caballero B, Cousins RJ, Tucker KL, Ziegler TR, editors. Modern Nutrition in Health and Disease. 11th ed. Baltimore, MD: Lippincott Williams & Wilkins; 2014. pp. 317-324

[32] Gibson GE, Blass JP. Thiamine-dependent processes and treatment strategies in neurodegeneration. Antioxidants & Redox Signaling. 2007;**9**:1605-1619

[33] McCormick DB. Thiamin. In: Shils ME, Young VR, editors. Modern Nutrition in Health and Disease. 6th ed. Philadelphia, PA: Lea & Febiger; 1988. pp. 355-361

[34] Bailey AL et al. Thiamin intake, erythrocyte transketolase (EC 2.2.1.1) activity and total erythrocyte thiamin in adolescents. British Journal of Nutrition. 1994;**72**:111-125

[35] Rivlin RS. Riboflavin. In: Coates PM, Betz JM, Blackman MR, et al., editors. Encyclopedia of Dietary Supplements. 2nd ed. Informa Healthcare: London and New York; 2010. pp. 691-699

[36] Said HM, Ross AC. Riboflavin. In: Ross AC, Caballero B, Cousins RJ, Tucker KL, Ziegler TR, editors. Modern Nutrition in Health and Disease. 11th ed. Baltimore, MD: Lippincott Williams & Wilkins; 2014. pp. 325-330

[37] Neugebauer J, Zanre Y, Wacker J. Riboflavin supplementation and

preeclampsia. International Journal of Gynaecology and Obstetrics. 2006;**93**:136-137

[38] Food and Nutrition Board. Dietary Reference Intakes for Thiamin, Riboflavin, Niacin, Vitamin B6, Folate, Vitamin B12, Pantothenic acid, Biotin, and Choline. Washington, DC: National Academy Press; 1998

[39] Penberthy WT, Kirkland JB. Niacin. In: Erdman JW, Macdonald IA, Zeisel SH, editors. Present Knowledge in Nutrition. 10th ed. Washington, DC: Wiley-Blackwell; 2012. pp. 293-306

[40] Kirkland JB. Niacin. In: Ross AC, Caballero B, Cousins RJ, Tucker KL, Ziegler TR, editors. Modern Nutrition in Health and Disease. 11th ed. Baltimore, MD: Williams & Wilkins; 2014. pp. 331-340

[41] MacKay D, Hathcock J, Guarneri. Niacin: Chemical forms, bioavailability, and health effects. Nutrition Reviews. 2012;**70**:357-366

[42] Miller JW, Rucker RB. Pantothenic acid. In: Erdman JW, Macdonald IA, Zeisel SH, editors. Present Knowledge in Nutrition. 10th ed. Washington, DC: Wiley-Blackwell; 2012. pp. 375-390

[43] Sweetman L. Pantothenic acid. In: Coates PM, Betz JM, Blackman MR, et al., editors. Encyclopedia of Dietary Supplements. 2nd ed. Informa Healthcare: London and New York; 2010. pp. 604-611

[44] Trumbo PR. Pantothenic acid. In: Ross AC, Caballero B, Cousins RJ, et al., editors. Modern Nutrition in Health and Disease. 11th ed. Baltimore, MD: Lippincott Williams & Wilkins; 2014. pp. 351-357

[45] Mackey A, Davis S, Gregory J. Vitamin B6. In: Shils M, Shike M, Ross A, Caballero B, Cousins R, editors. Modern Nutrition in Health and Disease. 10th ed. Baltimore, MD: Lippincott Williams & Wilkins; 2005

[46] Riggs KM, Spiro A 3rd, Tucker K, Rush D. Relations of vitamin B-12, vitamin B-6, folate, and homocysteine to cognitive performance in the normative aging study. The American Journal of Clinical Nutrition. 1996;**63**:306-314

[47] Herbert V. Vitamin B12 in Present Knowledge in Nutrition. 17th ed. Washington, DC: International Life Sciences Institute Press; 1996

[48] Herbert V, Das K. Vitamin B12 in Modern Nutrition in Health and Disease. 8th ed. Baltimore, MD: Williams & Wilkins; 1994

[49] Combs G. Vitamin B12 in the Vitamins. New York: Academic Press, Inc.; 1992

[50] Bailey LB, Caudill MA. Folate. In: Erdman JW, Macdonald IA, Zeisel SH, editors. Present Knowledge in Nutrition. 10th ed. Washington, DC: Wiley-Blackwell; 2012. pp. 321-342

[51] Institute of Medicine. Food and Nutrition Board. Dietary Reference Intakes: Thiamin, Riboflavin, Niacin, Vitamin B6, Folate, Vitamin B12, Pantothenic Acid, Biotin, and Choline. Washington, DC: National Academy Press; 1998

[52] Scott JM, Weir DG. Folate/vitamin B12 interrelationships. Essays in Biochemistry. 1994;**28**:63-72

[53] Gershoff SN. Vitamin C (ascorbic acid): New roles, new requirements? Nutrition Reviews. 1993;**51**:313-326

[54] Rebouche CJ. Ascorbic acid and carnitine biosynthesis. American Journal of Clinical Nutrition. 1991;**54**(Suppl):S1147-S1152

[55] McCormick DB, Zhang Z. Cellular assimilation of water-soluble vitamins

in the mammal: Riboflavin, B6, biotin and C. Proceedings of the Society of Experimental Biology and Medicine. 1993;**202**:265-270

[56] Bates CJ. Bioavailability of vitamin C. European Journal of Clinical Nutrition. 1997;**51**(Suppl 1):S28-S33

[57] Kareem MM, Baqir SJ, Aowda SA, Hussein FA. Determination of vitamin C (ascorbic acid) concentration in some of commercial products, by redox titration. UOB Journal of Pure & Applied Sciences. 2010;**3**:18

[58] Kareem MM. Chemistry of Fruits. Jordan: DAR SAFA Publishing-Distributing; 2020. ISBN: 978-9923-28-014-0

Chapter 4

Malnutrition: Current Challenges and Future Perspectives

Joseph Kiprop Choge

Abstract

Achievement of good nutrition is important in Universal Healthcare; hence, all stakeholders should be updated regarding management of malnutrition and challenges encountered, especially in resource-constrained societies of the world. Coexistence of multiple predisposing factors of malnutrition therefore compounds its diagnosis and management. It is of paramount importance therefore that the vulnerable population should be provided with adequate knowledge to alleviate the nutritional challenges they encounter. Capacity building of the healthcare personnel that are entrusted to serve such vulnerable societies should be improved appropriately. Healthy nutrition policy makers, implementers, and evaluators in all healthcare sectors should be conversant with new developments in management of malnutrition and challenges including those encountered in case studies, such as one recently encountered in Kenya, during the management of isoniazid induced pellagra (IPT) in a TB patient also on antiretroviral therapy. Food fortification, nixtamalization, provision of ready-to-use therapy foods (RUTFs), and innovative lipid-based nutrient supplements are relatively new areas whose nutrition policy makers, implementers, and evaluators should be well updated in. As part of nutrition optimization among those at risk, the nonadherence to exclusive breastfeeding for at least 6 months, which globally remains unacceptably high (59%), should urgently be addressed through appropriate and widespread counseling.

Keywords: breastfeeding, challenges, counseling, fortification, innovative lipid-based nutrient supplements, malnutrition, nixtamalization, nutrition, optimization, universal healthcare

1. Introduction

Malnutrition has been clearly described by the World Health Organization, among other entities dealing with the professional aspects of the subject matter [1, 2]. The nutritional imbalance can be classified in various ways, especially for purposes of proper and adequate management. Currently, the categories of malnutrition include undernutrition, overweight, and obesity, among others that will be substantiated shortly. The study of malnutrition, especially in developing countries, will remain important for a long time to come. This is because vulnerable communities, families, and/or individuals therein are likely to be adversely affected, with consequences of morbidity and mortality. Significantly large proportions (about 50%) of children aged five and below die from malnutrition and its complications, including infections. The severity, prevalence, and incidence of such infections may delay recuperation. Stunted growth and impaired cognitive and other aspects of child development may adversely affect learning of children during their first few years (more so the first 1000 days of life).

2. Worrying global prevalence trends of malnutrition

According to 2019 statistics from the World Health Organization and UNICEF [1–3], malnutrition is cosmopolitan, and its prevalence remains unacceptably high, consequently impacting negatively on the lives of the affected children. Approximately one third of women of reproductive age had anemia, while obesity affected a slightly higher proportion (39%) of the world's adult population. Underweight babies constitute a further 20 million, despite a noted slow decline in stunted growth. In 2018, just over a fifth (21.9%) of the world's children aged five had stunted growth, despite its overall global prevalence decline from 32.5% during the period between the years 2000 and 2018. During the same period, the population of stunted children decreased in terms of millions (from 198.2 to 149.0). Of this proportion, nearly 40% lived in South Asia, and a similar proportion lived in Africa south of Sahara (SSA), although an alarming proportional increase has been noted from west and central Africa (22.4 million to 28.9 million). Earlier in 2010, 49 million children aged five and below were wasted, while a further 17 million suffered from severe wasting thus translating to 7.3 and 2.4%, respectively. One worrying global trend is the fact that about 45% of mortality among children aged five and below is linked to malnutrition, the bulk of these occurring in low- and middle-income countries. A further global trend is that 528 million (29%) of reproductive-age women are vulnerable to anemia occasioned by inadequate dietary iron supplementation. In the low and middle - income Countries, the rates of childhood obesity and overweight were on the rise, estimated to nearly threefold rise in prevalence during the period between the years 2000 and 2018 alone, in Eastern Europe, Central Asia, the Middle East, and Northern Africa. The prevalence in these regions ranges between 8.8 and 11.2%, respectively. Eastern and south-east Asia, the Pacific, and northern Africa account for more than a third of the world's overweight children. The gender distribution of these statistics tends to show higher stunting rates among boys than girls. This is thought to be due to the fact that boys have relatively higher risk of low birth weight and preterm birth than girls. These disparities were noted to be prevalent in Latin America, South-ease Asia, and the Caribbean. More attention should then be placed on these regions by those dealing with intervention measures. WHO [3] report also cites that those who are at risk of malnutrition include infants, children, women, and adolescents and that optimization of nutrition early in life (specifically within the first 1000 days of life) will ensure the child gets the best possible start in life with its life-long benefits. Unfortunately, the nonadherence to the recommended prevalence of breastfeeding practices among many societies of the world remains relatively low and worrying, since only 41% (hence 59% non-compliance) of infants aged 6 months or less were exclusively breastfed and only 45% were continually breastfed for at most 2 years in 2017 [4].

3. Factors contributing to good nutrition

Before we consider the factors that predispose to malnutrition, let us first discuss the factors that contribute to good nutrition. These factors play an important role, especially in places where the resources are inadequate for the affected society and/or families [5]. Many of these factors are intertwined, especially in developing countries, where small-scale subsistence farming is practiced. The most notable of these are good agricultural practices, good and vibrant economy, healthy enabling environment, healthy social and family life, good antenatal and perinatal care, and early screening and control of preventable diseases. We shall now revisit each of these factors.

3.1 Good agricultural practices

Parents and household heads need to take responsibility in ensuring good agricultural practices (especially clearing farm land at the right time, planting sufficient good crops, using irrigation and fertilizer where necessary, getting appropriate advice from agricultural extension workers, harvesting at the right time, and safe storing the food to avoid losses through pests, a good transport and distribution system to get enough good food to all regions) are done appropriately. Chronic and irresponsible alcoholism by those charged with providing for the family, for example, may lead to poor (or inadequately productive) agricultural practices that will lead to loss of family income, poverty, and family neglect and may lead to malnutrition, among other health challenges in the family. Improvement of nutrition and prevention of malnutrition require energetic and cooperative efforts directed toward all these factors.

3.2 Good and vibrant economy

Those in influential leadership and governance of societies should on priority basis ensure there is a good economy in place. This should guarantee sufficient resources allocated to support adequate food and fuel/energy, health and education, and good education, among other society needs. Unfortunately, this is not always the case in many parts of the world, especially in developing countries.

3.3 Healthy enabling environment

Each country should ensure there is equitable availability and distribution of safe and sufficient water for drinking, cooking, cleaning, and other uses. Environmental sanitation and sewage treatment and management should also be appropriate. If this kind of environment is lacking, then the affected society will be vulnerable to many health problems, including related nutrition challenges.

3.4 Good education

Provision of appropriate and adequate knowledge on good nutrition and child health to the societies is critical. In most developing countries, this can effectively be done by those charged with the responsibility of disseminating such knowledge to schools, families, and any other modes of communication to large populations. Through good health education, the right attitudes and practices that promote good nutrition to the most vulnerable groups (especially children and mothers) will be guaranteed.

3.5 Healthy social and family life

Dissemination of adequate knowledge on family planning matters, at the right time to the right audience, is important. The right size of and the availability of adequate resources to the family and the presence of a health social environment in a family are paramount. This will ensure adequacy of food and attention to the whole family, especially younger children who usually need more care. Arrangements to ensure adequate resources for food, shelter, and other needs are maintained even if either or both parents have to work and a caretaker has to look after the children in their absence. Good supervision to ensure children get adequate and appropriate food should be in place at all times (at home, in day-care centers, and other such places); otherwise, some children might become malnourished. Care for children from broken or incomplete families directly affects nutritional status, especially if the social integration and communal care are lacking.

3.6 Good antenatal and perinatal care

Pregnant mothers require good antenatal care, especially to ensure good nutrition during pregnancy in order to avoid giving birth to low birth weight babies and to prevent intrauterine growth retardation and prematurity.

3.7 Early screening and control of preventable diseases

Immunization and vaccinations done appropriately at the right time to the right people will ensure early detection and prevention of diseases. Early screening for congenital malformations that interfere with child's eating or food utilization (such as cleft lip/palate, congenital hypertrophic pyloric stenosis) can alleviate related health problems and their management.

4. Factors predisposing to malnutrition

Globally, inadequate food intake is the most common cause of malnutrition: [5, 6]. In developing countries, inadequate food intake may be due to poverty, insufficient, or inappropriate food supplies or early weaning and premature stopping of breastfeeding. Ignorance about the need to have a balanced diet (and lack of adequate knowledge about the appropriate food and the right quantities needed by each family member) and ignorance about the importance of breastfeeding may be important contributing factor(s) in some places, especially if those endowed with the responsibility of disseminating the right knowledge fail to do it appropriately. Psychosocial issues, such as premature death of a breastfeeding mother, deliberate maternal deprivation from whatever reason may also contribute to childhood malnutrition. Single mothers (due to death of a spouse, separation, or divorce) may also face the challenge of premature stoppage of breastfeeding, owing to the fact that such mothers have to constantly provide food and other needs for the family, without the help of a spouse. This challenge might also contribute to maternal deprivation of adequate food to the baby, abuse of the rights toward the baby, especially if the baby was born out of unplanned pregnancy. The introduction of breast milk banks has alleviated this problem in certain places, but adequate health education of the safety and convenience of this approach has not yet been fully embraced culturally by many societies. The fear of disease transmission through breast milk remains a hindrance of new approaches of providing breast milk to babies whose mothers are missing or are not able to produce enough breast milk. In some areas, cultural and religious food customs may play a role. For example, ignorance of what constitutes a balanced diet can contribute to malnutrition. Consequently, certain families might sell most food sources they produce and actually need for the family, in order to buy larger quantities of food supplies they do not actually need. Poor family planning is a major problem in some cultures, especially where polygamy and bearing many children are encouraged, without due regard to limited available resources to support the families. Poor personal and environmental hygiene, due to inadequate sanitation, may aggravate situation by encouraging food contamination during food handling, preparation, and consumption. Consequently, the affected individuals will suffer from inherent risks of dangerous infectious diseases that will increase nutritional losses and/or altered metabolic demands. This scenario is likely to lead to repeated infections if the infrastructure lacks well-maintained sewage and sanitation facilities and/or supply of adequate clean water. Constant or frequent exposure to infection/infestation with intestinal and other worms such as hook worms and fish tape worms, among others will also predispose to nutritional iron deficiency anemia. Many people living under deplorable health conditions will also be exposed to many other parasites, including ascariasis, which contribute to food deprivation.

Chronic disease conditions and illnesses are important etiological factors of malnutrition: [5, 6]. This is especially more so in developed countries. People with chronic illnesses (especially children) are at relatively higher risk of nutritional problems. Some of the contributing factors include the following: chronic illnesses are frequently associated with loss of appetite and therefore intake of inadequate food. Some chronic illnesses are also associated with increased metabolic demands, hence increasing caloric needs. Any chronic illness that adversely affects the liver, pancreas, or intestines has the potential of adversely impairing food digestion and absorption. Other chronic illnesses that are associated with malnutrition include surgical diseases (such as cleft lip and/or palate, chronic hypertrophic pyloric stenosis), malignancies, congenital heart diseases, chronic renal failure, chronic bowel inflammatory diseases (such as ulcerative colitis), neuromuscular diseases, and cystic fibrosis, among others. Furthermore, risk of nutritional deficiency may be due to prematurity, failure to thrive for whatever cause, and exposure to toxins *in utero* (e.g., alcohol intake during pregnancy).

People with multiple food allergies (especially children) may become malnourished, due to challenges of dietary restrictions: [5, 6]. People with active allergic symptoms may have increased calorie and protein needs. This is partly because their state of morbidity predisposes them to lack of appetite during the time of ill-health and therefore without extra dietary supplements they might become malnourished. Furthermore, the allergy to certain foods denies them the benefit of the nutrients found in the food they are allergic to. If there is lack of appropriate dietary substitute, then the affected individuals will become malnourished with time.

5. Classification of malnutrition

Malnutrition can be classified into different categories [3, 7], namely, undernutrition, overnutrition, micronutrient-related malnutrition, severe acute (SAM), moderate acute (MAM), and global acute malnutrition (GAM), respectively. The assessment of body mass index (BMI) is one of the major ways of differentiating some of these categories. Details of BMI will be given later in the chapter.

Undernutrition consists of stunting, wasting, underweight, and micronutrient deficiencies. Stunting refers to a situation whereby children have a lower than normal height-for-age. Wasting refers to lower than normal weight-for-height, while underweight refers to lower than normal weight-for-age. Micronutrient deficiency refers to inadequate intake of vitamins and minerals. In more technical terms, the World Health Organization [3] defines these terms as follows. Underweight is defined as weight for age < -2 standard deviations (SD) of the WHO Child Growth Standards median. Stunting is defined as height for age < -2 SD of the WHO Child Growth Standards median. Wasting is defined as weight for height < -2 SD of the WHO Child Growth Standards median. The predisposing factors to some of these are known. Low birth weight is associated with intrauterine growth retardation or restriction, prematurity, or both. This situation is likely to ultimately predispose to poor health in the vulnerable societies. These situations, in addition to aggravating growth and cognitive and chronic disease development in adulthood, also predispose to morbidity and mortality, especially of neonates. Low-birth-weight infants are 20 times more likely to die of these than healthier infants.

Overnutrition comprises obesity and overweight. These are important because they are increasingly associated with lifestyle disorders, notably diabetes mellitus and cardiovascular diseases capable of complicating to stroke and even cancer that are responsible for morbidity and mortality from noncommunicable diseases. In more technical terms, overweight is defined as weight for height $> +2$ SD of the WHO Child Growth Standards median. Whereas undernutrition is prevalent among societies with inadequate food and the other predisposing factors already described, overnutrition is conversely associated with more affluent societies who tend to live more sedentary lives and can afford more palatable and fast-prepared junk food. These types of food stuffs are relatively cheap and readily available to a large section of the world population. No wonder the upsurge in related nutritional disorders. Variations in nutritional status may also be seen in individual families in a given community.

Micronutrient-related malnutrition occurs due to inadequate intake of vitamins and minerals. Micronutrients enable the body to produce enzymes, hormones, and other essential substances needed for proper growth and development of the human body. Among the micronutrients most essential are iodine, vitamin A, and iron. The deficiency of these micronutrients paused major health threats especially among children and pregnant women from low socioeconomic status.

The following categories are mainly for purposes of management of malnutrition [8]. Moderate acute malnutrition (MAM) refers to weight-for-height z-score (WHZ) between -2 and -3 or mid-upper arm circumference (MUAC) between 115 and <125 mm. Severe acute malnutrition (SAM) refers to WHZ < -3 or MUAC <115 mm, or the presence of bilateral pitting edema, or both. Global acute malnutrition (GAM) refers to the combination of MAM and SAM and is used as a measurement of nutritional status at a population level and as an indicator of the severity of an emergency situation. The prevalence thresholds for severity of malnutrition among children aged five and below are described elsewhere [5, 9–11].

6. Historical background and importance of classifying malnutrition

Part of the documented historical background of the classifications of malnutrition dates back to 1956, when Gómez and Galvan studied the factors they thought were associated with death among malnourished children Mexico City [12]. Initially, this classification was based on first, second, and third degrees, respectively [13]. The degrees were based on weight below a specified percentage of median weight for age [9] According to this classification, the risk of death increases with increasing degree of malnutrition [13]. An adaptation of Gomez's original classification is still used today. Whereas this modification provides a way of comparing malnutrition within and between populations, this classification has been criticized as too arbitrary and does not consider overweight as a classification of malnutrition, apart from the fact that height alone may not be the best indicator of malnutrition. Children who are born prematurely may be considered short for their age even if they have good nutrition [14]. Nevertheless, the criticism led to the establishment of a new classification of malnutrition by John Conrad Waterlow [15]. Waterlow classification therefore combines weight-for-height (indicating acute episodes of malnutrition) with height-for-age to show the stunting that results from chronic malnutrition [16]. One advantage of the Waterlow classification over the Gomez classification is the fact that weight for height can be examined even if ages are not known [15]. The World Health Organization has since modified some of these classifications [9].

7. Importance of malnutrition classification in children

Stunting, wasting, underweight, and overweight indicators are important for assessing nutritional imbalance resulting in undernutrition among children, according to the World Health Organization [12]. As far as child growth is concerned, it is internationally recognized as an important indicator of health in populations. It is also important as indicator for nutritional status. The cumulative effects of malnutrition and the consequent complications among children are reflected by the percentages of children with stunting (low height for age) from and even before birth. The degree of stunting can therefore be interpreted as an indicator for the existence of poor environmental conditions that have the potential of restricting child growth. The proportion of underweight and/or wasted children also indicates acute weight loss, stunting, or both. Hence, it may be difficult to interpret 'underweight' because it is a composite indicator. Thus, underweight, even in its mildest form, indicates increased risk of childhood mortality, and this risk increases among severely underweight children. Inadequate food and recurrent childhood infections also have a tendency to increase the risk of mortality among affected children. Stunting predisposes to poor child performance in school and also to delayed developmental milestones and decreased intellectual development in terms of capacity. Childhood wasting also predisposes to immunosuppression, subsequently leading to increased susceptibility to infections.

Childhood obesity may precede the same in adulthood. Overweight and obesity (especially in adolescence and childhood) increase the risk of developing short- or long-term health problems, notably cardiovascular disorders and diabetes mellitus. Also, among the risks are musculoskeletal disorders (e.g., osteoarthritis) and malignancies of the breast, colon, and/or endometrium. The assessment of nutritional status of a given population is an important indicator for moderate and/or severe malnutrition.

8. Importance of malnutrition classification in women

Chronic malnutrition may adversely affect the growth of bones in girls, such that those affected are likely to have abnormal short stature, with relatively smaller pelvis than women with normal growth. Thus, the affected women may get complications during child birth, which might cause obstructed labor that might be dangerous for the baby, the mother, or both. Other birth-related complications of such mothers include the birth of babies with lower weight than normal (low birth weight babies), retarded intrauterine growth, and short stature later in adult life. Their likely general maternal morbidity may also adversely affect quality of healthcare of the mother and baby during pregnancy.

8.1 Anthropometric measurements

The major mode of assessment of nutritional status of gravid women and children is by the use of anthropometry (the process by which anthropometric measurements are serially taken). The measurements have been developed and improved over time. These measurements taken quantitatively and involve measurements of muscle girth, bulk, and sometimes muscle power and tone if other inherent nervous system problems are suspected. Bone length and density as well as quantity of adipose tissue may also be measured. However, the main anthropometric measurements are those of weight and height, and from these two, the body mass index (BMI) may be calculated. Also important are the measurements of head circumference, waist, hip, and limb circumferences as well as the thickness of skin folds. As already discussed in the previous section, such measurements are important in assessing the nutritional status of children and pregnant mothers. For children, the individual measurements done, respectively, determine whether or not each child is normally growing, is stunted, is wasted, or is underweight. For pregnant women, the measurements will determine timely interventions of correcting the malnutrition and even the mode of delivery (normal or assisted vaginal delivery or by Cesarean section). The measurement will therefore also determine the place and cost of delivery if specialists may be required during and after delivery. The type of nutritional follow up will also be determined by the serial quantitative anthropometric measurements. In more sophisticated healthcare set-ups such as in developed countries [17–19], anthropometry is not only vital for timely and appropriate diagnosis of abnormalities such as microcephaly, macrocephaly, anencephaly, diabetes mellitus, hypertension, and other lifestyle-related illnesses, but it also enables early diagnosis of metabolic syndrome and dyslipidemia, among others. Furthermore, the measurements are helpful in initial assessment and progress of physical fitness of athletes and even the general population [18, 19] and for monitoring of nutritional status of children and pregnant mothers [20, 21] by the use of newer scientific methods in comparison to conventional ones.

However, there are situations whereby such measurements are discouraged. These include individuals who have undergone limb amputation or those with Plaster of Paris. Anthropometric measurements may be erroneous for those with gross abdominal obesity because of difficulties of locating important reference bony landmarks. Inexperienced personnel taking the measurements may also increase the chances of erroneous measurements.

The body mass index (BMI, which is the weight in kilograms divided by the square of the height in meters—kg/m^2) is helpful in determining the classification of obesity, overweight, or underweight in both children and adults. The range of measurements calculated in this manner, in relation to given limits for the normal and abnormal values, will determine whether or not an individual is healthy in terms of BMI. Normal weight BMI range is generally between 18.5 and 24.9. Moderate to severe thinness in adults is indicated by BMI < 17.0, whereas a BMI < 18.5 is an indication of underweight. Individuals considered overweight are those with BMI ≥ 25.0, while those considered obese have BMI ≥ 30.0. The health implications of underweight, obesity, and overweight have already been discussed in the previous section. Generally, overweight and obesity predispose to a wide range of noncommunicable diseases. Among these are malignancies of various types, musculoskeletal and respiratory disorders, gallbladder diseases, ischemic (coronary) heart disease, and associated complications such as heart attack and stroke, among others. Some of these drastically reduce the lifespan and/or quality of life of affected individuals. The significance and implications of BMI are therefore of paramount importance in public health, which cannot be anymore overemphasized.

8.2 Pathophysiology of malnutrition

Malnutrition and its complications may affect virtually part of the human body basically because the energy provided by various biomolecules, vitamins, and micronutrients is essential for all physiological and biochemical functions in the body [6, 22]. Dietary deficiency of these nutrients therefore adversely affects the functioning of the body. Digestion of protein to produce amino acids is required for metabolism, enzymatic functions, and antibody production, among others. Micronutrients are required as cofactors for various metabolic functions essential for the body. When nutritional deficiency occurs, the body is forced to readjust its hormonal secretion and metabolic functions (a process known as reductive adaptation) in order to economize on the available nutrients for survival.

Among the adjustments are reduced thyroxine and insulin productions to minimize metabolic rate and increase glucose availability for generation of energy, respectively. Consequently, protein deficiency leads to impaired/arrested or failed physical growth and/or cognitive development. Immunity may also be suppressed due to relatively reduced antibody production occasioned by protein deficiency. Other immune response changes include decreased complement system and certain cytokine functioning, impaired phagocytosis due to decreased T-lymphocyte levels, loss of delayed hypersensitivity, and decreased secretion of immunoglobulin A (IgA). These are subsequently associated with increased susceptibility to a wide variety of infections. Diarrhea from the infections may further aggravate the situation by causing anorexia, decreased nutrient absorption (also due to villous atrophy that occurs especially in kwashiorkor), and direct nutrient losses, among other changes requiring increased metabolic needs of the body. In order for the body to meet its energy demands, the body resorts to breaking down stored fat and muscles, resulting in body wasting seen especially in marasmus. Other pathological changes within the brain that have been confirmed in various studies, include reduced myelination, brain neurons, weight and growth rate, thinning of the cerebral cortex, and changes in the dendritic spines in severely malnourished infants. Fatty degeneration of the liver and the heart coupled by small bowel atrophy and decreased intravascular volume may result in secondary hyperaldosteronism in some. A differential diagnosis of these changes is severe mental retardation [22].

8.3 Clinical presentation of malnutrition

Protein energy malnutrition (PEM), sometimes synonymously described as undernutrition, commonly presents with a myriad of clinical symptoms and signs [6]. The complaints elicited during history taking typically include poor weight gain, slowing of linear growth, behavioral changes such as apathy (lack of interest in surroundings), irritability, anxiety, impaired social responsiveness, and some deficits in attention. Oedema, apathy, hair and skin changes, and reduction of subcutaneous tissue are frequently observable in patients with PEM [23], and the most affected are the face, arms, legs, and buttocks. It is not unusual to find coexistence of PEM with deficiency of micronutrients, especially in developing countries. The micronutrient-deficient individuals may actually present with features resembling those of PEM. Kwashiorkor and marasmus are two forms of PEM that commonly coexist (hence known as marasmic-kwashiorkor) or may be distinct as separate clinical entities [24]. PEM may cause cognitive impairment, especially if the nutritional deficiency occurs between the third trimester of pregnancy and the first 2 years of life [25]. Iron deficiency anemia in children aged 2 years and below is likely to affect brain function as an acute and probably also as a chronic occurrence.

Similarly, the deficiency of folic acid has also been associated with defective development of neural tubes.

'Kwashiorkor', which is a Ghanaian term that means 'the sickness the older one gets when the next sibling is born', is caused by inadequate consumption of dietary protein [24]. The descriptive definition rightly identifies the fact that the older sibling is deprived of breast feeding and instead is weaned on a diet composed largely of carbohydrates and devoid of proteins [26], thus rendering the older sibling malnourished. The clinical presentation of kwashiorkor mainly includes but exclusive to oedema, apathy, failure to thrive, underweight, and hair changes. Oedema occurs due to hypoalbuminemia following decreased oncotic pressure and consequent fluid extravasation to tissues. Oedema affects the face and the upper and lower extremities and may be slight or gross (anasarca), depending on the degree of protein deficiency. The presence of ascites and pleural effusion suggests the existence of peritoneal infection with tuberculosis (TB peritonitis). Failure to thrive (underweight, usually between 60 and 80% of expected body weight or failed growth) commonly occurs and may be masked by oedema, especially in lower extremities. Unlike in marasmus, kwashiorkor presents with muscle wasting (but with retention of subcutaneous tissue). Wasting of muscles is especially seen on chest, upper arms, and gluteal area. Children with high intake of carbohydrates (hence known as 'sugar babies') but with coexisting kwashiorkor tend to have generalized puffiness and much subcutaneous fat but no skin changes. Those affected also frequently have very low albumin levels. Close observation of an affected child will typically reveal apathy (due to mental changes, making the child apathetic and miserable; hence, the child may sit the whole day without interest in food or surroundings). This is in contrast with marasmus whereby the child is extremely wasted and hungry but may even be playful and interested in surroundings. Hair changes (altered texture, loss of luster, fine, straight, soft, scarce, and easily plucked hair with color changes ranging from brown, and reddish, to gray blond or white) are observable. Skin changes are also common, depicting pigmentation or depigmentation, desquamation (flunky-paint or irregular dermatoses), or ulceration. In severe cases of kwashiorkor, the skin may resemble extensive burns over the child's legs, buttocks, and perineum. Severe cases are prone to potentially fatal hypothermia, due to decreased basal metabolic rate (BMR); hence, the skin cannot respond to a fall in environmental temperature. Hypothermia victims may die especially at night when temperature is very low. Changes in mucous membranes include angular stomatitis, cheilosis, smooth tongue, perianal ulceration, and papillar atrophy. Hepatomegaly may occur due to fatty infiltration of the liver and also may occasion by profound but potentially fatal hypoglycemia. Gastrointestinal changes include anorexia, nausea, and vomiting. Diarrhea is nearly always profused and may result in dehydration and electrolyte imbalance. Dehydration is more chemical than infective in origin. If chemical (malabsorptive) diarrhea occurs, it causes decrease in enzymes, secondarily associated with villous atrophy (the atrophied portions are the tips where lactose is absorbed, hence resulting in lactose intolerance), low proteins, and pancreatic atrophy. Lactose intolerance may also occur and may be due to failure to absorb lactose, resulting in osmotic diarrhea. Lactose in the gut also predisposes to fermentation by normal gut flora, resulting in lactic acid formation, hypoperistalsis that may aggravate diarrhea. Anemia is frequently present and tends to display dimorphic (microcytic/macrocytic hypochromic) picture. If purpura and thrombocytopenia occur, they unfortunately indicate guarded/severe prognosis if no urgent management intervention is instituted.

'Marasmus' (which means 'to waste away') is caused by combined inadequate intake of protein and energy, which causes gaunt expression, severe wasting, leaving little or no edema, minimal subcutaneous fat, severe muscle wasting, and abnormally low serum albumin levels. Metabolism in such a child is adapted to prolonged survival [24, 27]. In contrast to the situation in kwashiorkor, muscle wasting in marasmus is associated with loss of subcutaneous tissue. Marasmus in some semiliterate societies is sometimes described as 'a child with an appearance of an old man wearing an oversized coat', for lack of better description to make it better understood by those very ignorant of the dangerous situation the child is in and requiring urgent intervention. The child's interest in surroundings and playful nature is therefore deceptive. Marasmus is typically seen in places with severe famine, conflict or war-torn areas with significant food restriction, or more severe cases of anorexia [24]. A child with marasmus may be anemic, but less so than kwashiorkor and hair changes are also fewer than in kwashiorkor. Tuberculosis and other secondary coinfections may occur and should therefore be sought carefully.

Complications of malnutrition include infections, hypothermia, hypoglycemia, anemia, dehydration, electrolyte imbalance, growth retardation/failure to thrive, and thrombocytopenia/disseminated intravascular coagulopathy (DIC), among others.

8.4 Micronutrients (vitamins, minerals, and trace elements) and their toxicities

Micronutrients (vitamins, minerals, and trace elements), in addition to essential fatty acids and amino acids [28, 29], are important for health. Fat-soluble vitamins are A, D, E, and K, while B and C are water-soluble vitamins. Fat-soluble vitamins have a higher potential for toxicity than do water-soluble vitamins, owing to their ability to accumulate in the body. The most toxic are those vitamins that contain iron, especially the following acute ingestions by affected children. In the context of nutrition, a mineral is a chemical element required as an essential nutrient by organisms to perform functions necessary for life [30, 31]. Since minerals are elements, they cannot be synthesized biochemically by living organisms but are obtained by plants from soil [32]. Human beings obtain most of their minerals from eating plants and animals or from drinking water [32]. The five major minerals in the human body are calcium, phosphorus, potassium, sodium, and magnesium [30, 33]. The rest of the elements (at least 20 of them) with specific biochemical body functions are sulfur, iron, chlorine, cobalt, copper, zinc, manganese, molybdenum, iodine, and selenium, which serve as structural and functional roles and electrolytes [30, 34]. The most abundant elements in the body are oxygen, hydrogen, carbon, and nitrogen. Calcium makes up to 99% of bones and teeth and making up about 1.5% of body weight. Phosphorus makes up about two thirds of calcium and about 1% of a person's body weight, while the other major minerals (sodium, potassium, chlorine, sulfur, and magnesium) constitute about 0.85% of the body weight. Overall, the 11 chemical elements (H, C, N, O, Ca, P, K, Na, Cl, S, and Mg) constitute 99.85% of the human body, with the rest forming only 0.15% of the human body [33]. The main sources and clinical presentation of micronutrient deficiencies and toxicities are hereby tabulated (**Table 1**).

8.5 Useful investigations

Laboratory studies are done based on information from a complete history and physical examination [6]. The most helpful laboratory studies in assessing malnutrition in a child are hematological studies and laboratory studies evaluating protein status. Hematological studies should include a complete blood count (CBC) with red blood cell (RBC) indices, serum electrolytes, sedimentation rate, urinalysis, culture, and a peripheral smear. The blood tests help to exclude anemia from various nutritional deficiencies, including iron, folic acid, and vitamin B-12

Micronutrient	Functions/sources	Clinical presentation of deficiency/ toxicity
Vitamin A (Retinol)	Pro-vitamin A plant carotenoids (mainly carrots), animal products (liver, milk, kidney, fish oil), fortified foods, and drug supplements. Aids in night vision, growth. Isotretinoin (Accutane) used for the treatment of severe forms of acne, is closely related to the chemical structure of vitamin A (hence similar pharmacology and toxicity)	**Vitamin A deficiency** presents with night blindness, xerophthalmia, poor growth, and hair changes. Birth defects (when taken during pregnancy), intracranial hypertension, depression, and suicidal ideation have been reported with isotretinoin. **In acute vitamin A toxicity**, some or all of the following may be present: nausea, vomiting, anorexia, irritability, drowsiness, altered mental status, abdominal pain, blurred vision, headache, muscle pain with weakness, seizures. **In chronic vitamin A toxicity,** some or all of the following may be present: anorexia, hair loss, dryness of mucus membranes, fissures of the lips, pruritus, fever, headache, insomnia, fatigue, irritability, weight loss, bone fracture [35], hyperlipidemia, hypercalcemia [36]. Anemia, bone and joint pains, diarrhea, menstrual abnormalities, epistaxis. Vitamin A may cause increased bone resorption and promote the development of osteoporosis. **Carotenemia** (excess vitamin A intake) has no adverse consequences because the conversion of carotenes to retinol is not sufficient to cause toxicity. Carotenemia is manifested by a yellow-orange coloring of the skin, primarily the palms of the hands and the soles of the feet. It differs from jaundice in that the sclerae remain white
Vitamin D (Cholecalciferol)	Dairy products, egg yolks, liver, and fish. It facilitates calcium absorption and mobilizes calcium from bone	**Vitamin D deficiency**: Poor growth, rickets, and hypercalcemia. Place patients with vitamin D toxicity on a low-calcium diet. Consider oral calcium disodium edetate to increase fecal excretion of calcium. In cases of severe hypercalcemia, patients may require hydration, diuretics, steroids
Vitamin E (tocopherol and tocotrienol)	Vegetable oil, nuts, sunflower, wheat, green leafy vegetables, fish. It is an antioxidant and free-radical scavenger in lipophilic environments. Storage of the vitamin occurs in adipose tissue, the liver, and muscle. Vitamin E may block absorption of vitamins A and K. It also decreases low-density lipoprotein (LDL) cholesterol level at doses more than 400 IU/day	Since vitamin E may block absorption of vitamin K, a nutritional assessment for vitamin K deficiency is useful in patients who present with bleeding and a prolonged prothrombin time (PT). The effects of **acute vitamin E toxicity** include nausea, gastric distress, abdominal cramps, diarrhea, headache, fatigue, easy bruising, and bleeding—prolonged PT and activated partial thromboplastin time (aPTT), inhibition of platelet aggregation, diplopia —at dosages as low as 300 IU, muscle weakness, creatinuria. **Chronic Vitamin E toxicity** effects include all of the above, as well as suppression of other antioxidants and increased risk of hemorrhagic stroke. Vitamin E supplementation was shown to increase the risk of prostate cancer in healthy men, in the Selenium and Vitamin E Cancer Prevention Trial (SELECT) [37]
Vitamin K (phytonadione)	Produced by intestinal bacteria (vitamin K-2) and is found in green, leafy vegetables; cow's milk; and soy oil (vitamin K-1).	Vitamin E can prolong the prothrombin time (PT) by inhibiting vitamin K–dependent carboxylase, although

Micronutrient	Functions/sources	Clinical presentation of deficiency/ toxicity
	Vitamin K-1 supplements are usually 2.5–10 mg. Phytonadione promotes liver synthesis of factors II, VII, IX, and X	administration of vitamin K corrects this. High doses of vitamin E increase the vitamin K requirement; coagulopathy can occur in patients who are deficient in vitamin K [38, 39] (concomitant use of vitamin E and anticoagulants can also increase the risk of bleeding complications) [38, 39]
Vitamin B	**Vitamin B-1** (thiamin): found in organ meats, yeast, eggs, and green, leafy vegetables. Vitamin B-1 supplements usually contain 50–500 mg of vitamin B-1 per tablet. This vitamin is a cofactor for pyruvate dehydrogenase in the Krebs cycle. The RDA is 1.5 mg (0.7 mg for children aged 1–4 years). **Vitamin B-2:** The RDA for vitamin B-2 (riboflavin) is 1.7 mg (0.8 mg for children aged 1–4 years). Supplements usually are 25–100 mg. **Vitamin B-3** (niacin) is found in green vegetables, yeast (pumpernickel bagels may contain 190 mg of niacin), animal proteins, fish, liver, and legumes. Supplements are usually 20–500 mg per tablet. Vitamin B-3 synthesis requires tryptophan. Niacin is converted to nicotinamide adenine dinucleotide (NAD) or nicotinamide adenine dinucleotide phosphate (NADP). NAD and NADP are coenzymes for dehydrogenase-type reactions. **Vitamin B-6** functions in protein and amino acid metabolism. Pyridoxine is the treatment of choice for isoniazid overdose. It is also used by bodybuilders, as well as for the treatment, with varying results, of the following [40]: premenstrual syndrome (PMS), Carpal tunnel syndrome, Schizophrenia, Childhood autism, Attention deficit hyperactivity disorder (ADHD). **Vitamin B-12** (cyanocobalamin), which requires an intrinsic factor for absorption, is found in milk products, eggs, fish, poultry, and meat. Supplements usually contain 25–250 mcg of the vitamin per tablet. Vitamin B-12 is a treatment of pernicious anemia and cyanide poisoning	In large doses, niacin decreases synthesis of LDL cholesterol level. The RDA is 20 mg (9 mg for children aged 1–4 years). Vitamin B-6 (i.e., pyridoxine) is found in poultry, fish, pork, grains, and legumes. Supplements usually are 5–500 mg per tablet
Vitamin C (ascorbic acid)	**Functions:** An antioxidant and reducing agent, its controversial uses include treatment of upper respiratory tract infections and cancer [41]. Supplements are usually 100–2000 mg per capsule. **Sources:** Vitamin C is found in citrus fruits and vegetables	Rebound scurvy (in infants born to women taking high doses), renal colic (nephrolithiasis), diarrhea nausea, hemolysis (if glucose-6-phosphate dehydrogenase (G6PD) deficiency is present), dental decalcification, increased estrogen levels, occult rectal bleeding
Folate (folic acid)	**Functions**: Decreases the risk of neural tube defects and may reduce serum homocysteine levels (which are a coronary artery disease risk factor). It may also have a therapeutic role as an adjuvant therapy for the treatment of methanol toxicity, since it enhances the elimination of formate. **Sources:** Folate is found in oranges and green, leafy vegetables	Glossitis, anemia (megaloblastic), and neural tube defects (in fetuses of women without folate supplementation)

Micronutrient	Functions/sources	Clinical presentation of deficiency/ toxicity
Iron	**Function**: Required for many proteins and enzymes, notably hemoglobin to prevent anemia. **Sources**: Meat, seafood, nuts, beans, dark chocolate	**Deficiency**: Iron deficiency anemia features: Fatigue, anemia, decreased cognitive function, headache, glossitis, and nail changes (koilonychia). **Toxicity**: Iron overload disorder (hemochromatosis) [42]
Iodine	**Functions**: Required for synthesis of thyroid hormones, thyroxine, and triiodothyronine and to prevent goiter. **Sources**: Seaweed (kelp or kombu), grains, eggs, iodized salt, saltwater fish	**Iodine deficiency**: Severe iodine deficiency results in goiter. Population effects of severe iodine deficiency, termed iodine deficiency disorders (IDDs), include endemic goiter, hypothyroidism, and cretinism, decreased fertility rate, increased infant mortality, and mental retardation. **Iodine excess**: Iodism, Hyperthyroidism. **Iodine toxicity**: Excessive iodine may cause hypothyroidism by feedback inhibition of thyroid hormone production and conversion of triiodothyronine (T3) to less active thyroxine (T4).
Zinc	**Functions**: Zinc is necessary for growth, DNA synthesis and normal taste perception. It also supports wound healing, immune function and reproductive health and testosterone production. **Sources**: Oysters, Red meat, poultry, seafood, whole grains, nuts and fortified cereals	**Deficiency**: Anemia, dwarfism, hepatosplenomegaly, hyperpigmentation and hypogonadism, acrodermatitis enteropathica, diminished immune response, poor wound healing. Symptoms/ signs: acne, eczema, xerosis, seborrheic dermatitis, or alopecia, oral ulceration, stomatitis, or white tongue coating. Rarely, angular cheilitis disturbed sense of smell and taste, night blindness, impaired immunity, diarrhea, anorexia; psychological disturbances: behavioral abnormalities, such as irritability, lethargy, and depression (due to impaired cognitive functions), delayed growth, teratogenic effects, hypogonadism, delayed puberty, and sexual maturity. **Toxicity**: nausea, vomiting, abdominal pain, diarrhea, flu-like malaise, lowering of good HDL cholesterol (increased risk of heart disease). Decreased taste function (hypogeusia), copper deficiency (associated with sideroblastic and iron deficiency anemia and neutropenia), immunity suppression
Copper	**Functions**: It helps maintain a healthy metabolism, promotes strong and healthy bones and ensures the nervous system works properly. Required component of many redox enzymes, including cytochrome c oxidase. **Sources**: Liver, seafood, oysters, nuts, seeds; some: whole grains, legumes	**Copper deficiency**: fatigue and weakness (due to iron deficiency anemia; also copper is required to generate ATP), frequent sickness (due to neutropenia), weak and brittle bones (osteoporosis), learning and memory difficulties (e.g., Alzheimer's disease), walking difficulties, increased sensitivity to cold, pallor and premature gray hair (due to melanin underproduction), vision loss. **Copper toxicity [33]**: nausea, vomiting (food or blood), diarrhea, stomach pain, black, "tarry" stools, headaches, dyspnea, cardiac arrhythmias, low blood pressure, coma, jaundice, kidney damage, liver damage
Magnesium	**Function**: Required for processing ATP and for bones, energy transfer, storage, and	**Deficiency:** Hypomagnesemia (earliest: neuromuscular and neuropsychiatric

Micronutrient	Functions/sources	Clinical presentation of deficiency/ toxicity
	use; protein, carbohydrate, and fat metabolism; maintenance of normal cell membrane function; and the regulation of parathyroid hormone (PTH) secretion. Systemically, lowers blood pressure and alters peripheral vascular resistance. **Sources**: Spinach, legumes, nuts, seeds, whole grains, peanut butter, avocado	disturbances, common being hyperexcitability, neuromuscular irritability, including tremor, fasciculations, tetany, Chvostek and Trousseau signs, and convulsions, apathy, muscle cramps, hyperreflexia, acute organic brain syndromes, depression, general weakness, anorexia, vomiting; osteoporosis, nephrolithiasis—urinary stones; diabetes mellitus often associated). **Toxicity/excess**: Hypermagnesemia (neuromuscular symptoms—deep tendon reflex attenuation, facial paresthesias, muscle weakness—especially respiratory, causing apnea; conduction system symptoms)
Phosphorus	**Functions**: A component of bones, cells, in energy processing, in DNA and ATP (as phosphate) and many other functions. **Sources**: Red meat, dairy foods, fish, poultry, bread, rice, oats. In biological contexts, usually seen as phosphate	**Deficiency:** Hypophosphatemia (most asymptomatic; severe/chronic forms have weakness, bone pain, rhabdomyolysis, and altered mental status). **Toxicity/excess:** Hyperphosphatemia (asymptomatic; may have hypocalcemia—muscle cramps, tetany, and perioral numbness or tingling; uremia—fatigue, shortness of breath, anorexia, nausea, vomiting; sleep disturbances)
Potassium [43]	**Function:** A systemic electrolyte and is essential in co-regulating ATP. **Sources:** fruits, vegetables, beans and nuts, sweet potato, tomato, Irish potato	**Deficiency:** Hypokalemia (features of underlying cause; weakness and fatigue; muscle cramps and pain (severe); worsening diabetes control or polyuria; palpitations; psychological symptoms (e.g., psychosis, delirium, hallucinations, depression); cardiac arrhythmias; respiratory failure). **Toxicity/excess:** Hyperkalemia: (asymptomatic; nonspecific; frank muscle paralysis, dyspnea, palpitations, chest pain, nausea or vomiting, paresthesias)
Sodium [44, 45]	**Function:** A systemic electrolyte and is essential in co-regulating ATP with potassium. **Sources:** Table salt (sodium chloride, the main source), sea vegetables, milk, and spinach	**Deficiency:** Hyponatremia: (nausea and malaise, mild reduction in the serum sodium, lethargy, decreased level of consciousness, headache, and (if severe) seizures and coma). **Toxicity/excess**: Hypernatremia (elderly, diabetic, inadequate care; lethargy, confusion, abnormal speech, irritability, seizures, nystagmus, myoclonic jerks, tachycardia, oliguria, weakness)
Chlorine [46, 47]	**Function:** Needed for production of hydrochloric acid in the stomach and in cellular pump functions. **Sources:** (with sodium): beans, lentils, dairy products, seafood, banana, prune, carrot, orange	**Deficiency:** Hypochloremia [fluid loss, dehydration, weakness/fatigue, dyspnea, diarrhea or vomiting (fluid loss)]. **Excess:** Hyperchloremia (fluid retention, hypertension, muscle weakness, spasms, or twitches, irregular heart rate, confusion, difficulty concentrating, and personality changes, numbness or tingling, seizures and convulsions)
Calcium [48, 49]	**Function:** Needed for muscle, heart and digestive system health, builds bone, supports synthesis and function of blood cells. **Sources:** Dairy products, eggs,	**Deficiency:** Hypocalcaemia (acute symptoms: multiple CVS effects causing syncope, chronic heart failure, and angina; neuromuscular symptoms: numbness,

Micronutrient	Functions/sources	Clinical presentation of deficiency/ toxicity
	canned fish with bones (salmon, sardines), green leafy vegetables, nuts, seeds, tofu, thyme	tingling, tetany, bronchospasms, dysphagia, voice changes (laryngospasms)). **Excess/toxicity:** Hypercalcemia (nausea, vomiting, alterations of mental status, abdominal or flank pain, constipation, lethargy, depression, weakness and vague muscle/ joint aches, polyuria, polydipsia, nocturia, headache, confusion)
Manganese [50–52]	**Functions:** A cofactor in enzyme functions; antioxidant properties in mitochondria; has role in metabolism of carbohydrates, amino acids, cholesterol & gluconeogenesis; formation of health cartilage & bone; increases collagen production (improved wound healing). **Sources:** Whole grains (cereals, brown rice), legumes, seeds, nuts, leafy vegetables, tea, coffee, pineapples, sweet potatoes	**Deficiency:** Manganese deficiency (characterized, more so in animals than humans, by impaired growth, impaired reproductive function, skeletal abnormalities, impaired glucose tolerance, and altered carbohydrate and lipid metabolism; humans develop bone demineralization, decreased serum cholesterol, rashes). **Toxicity/excess:** Manganism (psychiatric and motor disturbances from chronic exposure; neurological symptoms including: reduced response speed, irritability, mood changes, and compulsive behaviors; more protracted exposure produces idiopathic Parkinsonism-like disorder, Lou Gehrig's disease and multiple sclerosis)
Chromium [53–55]	**Function:** Chromium can improve insulin sensitivity and enhance protein, carbohydrate, and lipid metabolism, although its mechanisms of action and quantity needed not well-defined. **Sources:** Broccoli, grape juice (especially red), meat, whole grain products, processed meats, high-bran breakfast cereals, coffee, nuts, green beans, broccoli, spices, and some brands of wine and beer	**Deficiency:** Chromium deficiency (due to total parenteral intake/I-V fluids: symptoms and signs include severely impaired glucose tolerance, weight loss, peripheral neuropathy, and confusion). **Excess:** Chromium toxicity [**Acute exposure**: Intense G.I.T irritation/ ulceration and corrosion, epigastric pain, nausea, vomiting, diarrhea, vertigo, fever, muscle cramps, hemorrhagic diathesis, toxic nephritis, renal failure, intravascular hemolysis, circulatory collapse, liver damage, acute multisystem organ failure, and coma/death, depending on the dose (Hay, Derazon et al., 2000; Lewis, 2004; Meditext, 2005). **Chronic esxposure**: Repeated skin contact causes incapacitating eczematous dermatitis with edema; conjunctiva and mucous membrane irritation, nasal ulcers and perforations, keratitis, gingivitis, periodontitis and lung cancer (Cohen and Costa, 1998; Lewis, 2004; Meditext, 2005); bronchitis, sinusitis, nasal polyps; liver and kidney toxicities (Rom, 2007)]
Selenium [35, 40, 56, 57]	**Function**: Essential to activity of antioxidant enzymes like glutathione peroxidase. Also plays role in thyroid hormone metabolism, DNA synthesis, reproduction and protection from infection. **Sources**: Brazil nuts, Sea foods (especially fish—yellow-fin tuna fish, cod, red snapper, and herring), organ meats/ beef & poultry, grains, dairy products, eggs, rice, beans, whole-wheat bread	**Deficiency:** Selenium deficiency [characterized by male/female infertility, muscle weakness, fatigue, mental fog, alopecia, and weakened immunity). People at risk of deficiency: thyroid (goiter), dialysis, HIV, malignancy, Crohn's and Grave's disease patients, pregnancy]. **Excess:** Selenosis [characterized by diarrhea, fatigue, hair loss, joint pain, nail discoloration or brittleness and nausea. Symptoms persisting 90 days or longer

Micronutrient	Functions/sources	Clinical presentation of deficiency/ toxicity
		include fingernail discoloration and loss fatigue and hair loss]
Cobalt (cyanocobalamin) [58, 59]	**Functions:** Its part of vitamin B-12 (required in the synthesis of vitamin B-12; hence needed for erythropoiesis; also essential for maintaining the nervous system. Cobalt is also part of the biotin-dependent Krebs-cycle, for glucose/energy production. **Sources**: Animal products containing vitamin B-12 (milk products, eggs, fish, poultry, and meat)	**Deficiency:** Pernicious anemia (B-12 deficiency): numbness, Fatigue, and tingling sensation, later, decreased nerve function. **Excess:** Cobalt poisoning (characterized by toxic cardiomyopathy, polycythemia, leading to congestive cardiac failure). Poisoning can follow excessive inhalation, ingestion or direct body contact. It can also cause goiter or inactivity of thyroid and hyperglycemia. Cobalt poisoning has been reported after hip-replacement surgery if cobalt/ chromium was used during the surgery, as a metal-to-metal hip implant). Cobalt is contraindicated in people with Leber's syndrome, a rare eye condition, should not take it without medical advice; otherwise, it can result in blindness
Molybdenum [58]	**Functions**: It is a cofactor for several enzymes that breakdown xanthine, hypoxanthine, and sulfite. They also break down and detoxify many harmful compounds. It is affected by the amount of copper and sulfate in the diet. **Sources:** Legumes, whole grains (cereals), nuts, and leafy vegetables	**Deficiency:** Very rare. **Excess:** Molybdenum toxicity (gout-like syndrome, characterized by high levels of molybdenum, uric acid, and xanthine oxidase in blood). Molybdenum is contraindicated in patients with gallstones or kidney disease. Molybdenum supplements can cause a copper deficiency, by displacing copper from body tissues

Table 1.
Deficiencies and toxicities of micronutrients, including vitamins, minerals, and trace elements.

deficiencies, which are measured by assessing serum albumin, retinol-binding protein, prealbumin, transferrin, creatinine, and BUN levels. Others include retinol-binding protein, prealbumin, and transferrin determinations that are much better short-term indicators of protein status than albumin. A better parameter to use in the field is serum albumin, since it has a longer half-life. In children who have a history of adequate food intake and signs/symptoms of malnutrition, focus is made toward identifying the cause of malnutrition. Stool specimens should be obtained if the child has a history suggestive of presence of worms or other parasites or circumstances that predispose to malnutrition. Other useful tests include thyroid functions or sweat chloride tests, liver function and triglyceride tests (for suspected liver disease), zinc levels (especially if chronic diarrhea is present), blood and urine sugar levels (to rule out diabetes mellitus), and coeliac serology tests, among other tests, depending on suspected cause(s). Nutritional assessment parameters such as height and weight (for BMI), MUAC, head circumference in children aged three and below, and others that are recognized according to the WHO standards are also done.

8.6 Treatment and management principles and prevention of malnutrition

The principles laid down for the management of malnutrition are generally applied [6]. These include the need for multi-disciplinary professional approach for specific, supportive, and preventive management. Specific and supportive treatments will largely depend on the classification of malnutrition encountered, while preventive measures will also depend on avoiding the prevalent cause and the predisposing factors encountered by those affected. Specific treatments will focus on the actual cause(s) of the malnutrition diagnosed after thorough evaluation of history, physical examination, and various investigations. These include provision of specific dietary food measured out depending on their preparation or manufacture, in addition to appropriate food supplements that may be fortified or not, depending on the prevailing cultural and socioeconomic practices encountered. Supportive management entails the need to initially manage life-threatening anemia, hypoglycemia, and/or hypothermia if these are found. Zinc [60, 61], folic acid, iodine, and vitamins A and D, among other supplements may also be given if indicated. Any other micronutrient deficiencies must be corrected, especially for children who still require to growth and development. Prevention measures largely address the need to avoid the predisposing factors of malnutrition from recurring in future, through appropriate health education and follow-up assessment schedules and programs. Promotion of breastfeeding, appropriate weaning practices, and age-appropriate nutritional counseling are strongly recommended in developing countries where there are major challenges in getting safe alternatives for human milk. The need to address emerging trends of food fortification, Ready-to-Use Therapeutic Foods (RUFT) [62], and other related issues is also important. Supplementations that are beneficial for pregnant mothers worldwide need special appropriate attention [63, 64]. Nutritional researches, with a view to addressing emerging and/or re-emerging nutritional challenges, such as those associated with antiretroviral and pellagra (IPT) [65] should also be encouraged.

8.7 Food fortification and nixtamalization

Food fortification [66], described as the supplementation of one or more components to improve the benefits from the natural or artificial food products [67], has received much professional and cosmopolitan attention. Food fortification is either voluntary or mandatory. Voluntary fortification gives food manufacturers the option to add minerals, vitamins, or both, to the food to be fortified, provided there is compliance with the laid down rules and regulations by Food and Drug Administration (FDA). On the other hand, mandatory fortification provides no option to do the same, in order to ensure that the significant public health need(s) is/are addressed adequately. Some of the mandatory fortifications achieved in the past include that of global iodized salt, vitamins A and D, zinc, folic acid, and iron and fortification of several B vitamins (thiamin, riboflavin, and niacin) to baking flour in certain countries, such as the United States during the 1940s onward, among many others. Such approaches by the FDA have successfully seen the reduction of neural tube defects (by 1998) among other problems. Food fortification as the major approach to the treatment of malnutrition is considered more cost effective and enables improvement of health achievable over a relatively shorter time than other forms of food aid. Many countries continue to identify their own fortification requirements and the approaches to address them; hence, fortification programs should be developed in this manner to address other common nutritional deficiencies. Iron deficiency, among many others, still needs to be addressed locally and globally. Despite the progress in food fortification, there are still major challenges to be overcome to ensure that malnutrition is well managed. However, precautions need to be taken to avoid over-fortification, by ensuring that minimum and maximum daily dietary requirements for fortification are met for each type of fortification. To achieve these, global authorities, including the World Health

Organization among others that adhere to evidence-based data for such important decisions, should lead the way.

Although nixtamalization (the process for the preparation of maize/corn or other grain, by soaking and cooking them in an alkaline solution—usually lime water or wood ash lye then washed and hulled to soften them) is an ancient practice of improving the nutritional value of maize and other grains such as sorghum, some of its benefits (e.g., the ability to remove between 97 and 100% of aflatoxin from contaminated maize) [66] may continue to encourage the practice in places where maize is the staple food. The fact that pellagra was in the past found to be endemic in poor populations that used maize in southern parts of the United States during the early period of the twentieth century [68] does not rule out the possibility of the same happening in contemporary times within the developing world. It is encouraging to note that pellagra was nearly eliminated in the developed world after fortification of wheat flour was achieved [69]. However, it might remain a challenge in places where such fortification has not been fully achieved, a likely scenario in many developing countries. The fact is that case studies such as the one described in Kenya recently (although this was a patient on antiretroviral therapy and prone to drug induced pellagra on treatment for tuberculosis) [65] may suggest the need to explore the possibility of existing pellagra due to niacin deficiency and in the absence of nixtamalization—a process that is rarely practiced in some societies, despite the need for it in some. In this regard perhaps, nixtamalization may still have a place in modern societies, especially in the developing world, and may need to be explored and improved. This has in the past been done with some benefits of reducing pellagra, improving availability of dietary calcium, copper, and zinc and removal of mycotoxins (aflatoxin) that is produced by *Fusarium proliferatum* and *Fusarium verticillioides* in certain places [70]. However, other unexplored effects (beneficial and adverse) may need to be investigated through further research.

8.8 Innovative lipid-based nutrient supplements and ready-to-use therapeutic foods (RUTF)

In addition to food fortification already described, innovative lipid-based nutrient supplements have also been introduced to alleviate undernutrition in vulnerable populations (notably infants, lactating mothers, and pregnant women). The project has already been piloted in several countries, including Burkina Faso, Ghana, and Malawi, among others. Some of their products had already been fortified by 2011 [71], namely, micronutrient powder (MNP) and lipid-based nutrient supplements (LNS); these are effective in reducing anemia and iron deficiency. Both are designed to be easily consumable by infants (thus advantageous over the pill forms commonly prepared as micronutrient pill supplements). However, an evaluation study [72] suggested that the micronutrients constituted in it may alone be insufficient to stimulate linear growth. Many studies (especially on LNS) applicable to different cultural settings are ongoing, despite challenges associated with adding micronutrients into the product.

Also introduced for better management of malnutrition are Ready-to-Use Therapeutic Foods (RUTF), which are high-energy lipid-based spreads that are designed to be used for the treatment of severe acute malnutrition (SAM) and in any cultural setting [62, 73]. F-75 and F-100 are two commonly available formulations from the World Health Organization (WHO) [74], which are used for the management of severe acute malnutrition. Their preparation process is elaborate [62], and the products are highly successful in terms of affordability and availability, in the management of malnutrition in various healthcare settings [73]. They are recommended by the World Health Organization and should gradually introduce until the child attains normal growth [75, 76]. Some have been successfully used in African countries, especially among children aged 5 years and below [67]. Like all other new formulations, the current and future challenges that RUTF may have should to be considered especially those concerning their safety, reliability, and affordability with short- and/or long-term use.

Author details

Joseph Kiprop Choge
Department of Clinical Medicine, University of Kabianga, Kenya

*Address all correspondence to: jchoge@kabianga.ac.ke

References

[1] Mehta NM, Corkins MR, Lyman B, Malone A, Goday PS, Carney LN, et al. Defining pediatric malnutrition: A paradigm shift towards etiology-related definitions. Journal of Parenteral and Enteral Nutrition. 2013;**37**(4):460-481

[2] WHO. Malnutrition—The Global Picture. World Health Organization. Available from: http://www.who.int/home-page/

[3] UNICEF/WHO/World Bank Joint Child Malnutrition Estimates. March 2019 edition.

[4] United Nations Children's Fund. Data. Infant and young child feeding. Available from: https://data.unicef.org/topic/nutrition/infant-and-young-child-feeding/

[5] Bwibo N, Stanfield P, et al. Child health. In: A Manual for Medical and Health Workers in Health Centres and Rural Hospitals. Nairobi: AMREF; 2005

[6] Shashidhar HR, Bhatia J, et al. Malnutrition. Medscape website. 2017

[7] Black RE, Laxminarayan R, Temmerman M, et al., editors. Reproductive, Maternal, Newborn, and Child Health: Disease Control Priorities. 3rd ed. Vol. 2. Washington, DC: The International Bank for Reconstruction and Development/The World Bank; 2016

[8] Alcoba G, Kerac M, Breysse S, Galetto-Lacour C, Salpeteur A, et al. Do children with uncomplicated severe acute malnutrition need antibiotics? A systematic review and meta-analysis. PLoS One. 2013;**8**(1):E53184

[9] Grover Z, Ee LC. Protein energy malnutrition. Pediatric Clinics of North America. 2009;**56**(5):1055-1068. DOI: 10.1016/j.pcl.2009.07.001

[10] IAP Textbook of Pediatrics. 4th ed. Vol. 1. New Delhi: Jaypee Publishers. pp. 143-144

[11] de Onis M et al. Prevalence thresholds for wasting, overweight and stunting in children under 5 years. Public Health Nutrition. 2018;**22**(1):1-5

[12] World Health Organization. Nutrition Landscape Information System (NLIS) Country Profile Indicators. 2010

[13] Stevenson RD, Conaway MR. Weight and mortality rates: "Gomez Classification" for children with cerebral palsy? Pediatrics. August 2011; **128**(2):e436-e437. DOI: 10.1542/peds.2011-1472

[14] Gueri M, Gurney JM, Jutsum P. The Gomez classification. Time for a change? Bulletin of the World Health Organization. 1980;**58**(5):773-777

[15] Waterlow JC. Classification and definition of protein-calorie malnutrition. British Medical Journal. 1972;**3**(5826):566-569. DOI: 10.1136/bmj.3.5826.566

[16] Watts G. John Conrad Waterlow. The Lancet. 2010;**376**(9757):1982. DOI: 10.1016/S0140-6736(10)62252-0

[17] Smits MM, Boyko EJ, Utzschneider KM, Leonetti DL, McNeely MJ, Suvag S, et al. Arm length is associated with type 2 diabetes mellitus in Japanese-Americans. Diabetologia. 2012;**55**(6): 1679-1684

[18] Vasconcelos AP, Cardozo DC, Lucchetti AL, Lucchetti G. Comparison of the effect of different modalities of physical exercise on functionality and anthropometric measurements in community-dwelling older women. Journal of Bodywork and Movement Therapies. 2016;**20**(4):851-856

[19] Kidy FF, Dhalwani N, Harrington DM, Gray LJ, Bodicoat DH, Webb D, et al. Associations between anthropometric measurements and cardiometabolic risk factors in White European and South Asian adults in the United Kingdom. Mayo Clinic Proceedings. 2017;**92**(6):925-933

[20] Hiremath R, Ibrahim J, Prasanthi K, Reddy HT, Shah RS, Haritha C. Comparative study of ultrasonographic and anthropometric measurements of regional adiposity in metabolic syndrome. Journal of Clinical and Diagnostic Research. 2017;**11**(8): TC01-TC05

[21] Gabbett T, Georgieff B. Physiological and anthropometric characteristics of Australian junior national, state, and novice volleyball players. Journal of Strength and Conditioning Research. 2007;**21**(3): 902-908

[22] Benitez-Bribiesca L, De la Rosa-Alvarez I, Mansilla-Olivares A. Dendritic spine pathology in infants with severe protein-calorie malnutrition. Pediatrics. 1999; **104**(2):e21

[23] Balint JP. Physical findings in nutritional deficiencies. Pediatric Clinics of North America. 1998;**45**(1):245-260

[24] Katsilambros N. Clinical Nutrition in Practice. John Wiley & Sons; 2011. p. 37. ISBN: 978-1-4443-4777-7

[25] Laus MF, Duarte Manhas Ferreira Vales L, Braga Costa TM, Sousa Almeida SO. Early postnatal protein-calorie malnutrition and cognition: A review of human and animal studies. International Journal of Environmental Research and Public Health. 2011;**8**(2):590-612. DOI: 10.3390/ijerph8020590

[26] Stanton J. Listening to the Ga: Cicely Williams' discovery of Kwashiorkor on the Gold Coast. Clio Medica: Studies in the History of Medicine and Health. 2001;**61**:149-171

[27] Chowdhury MSI, Akhter N, Haque M, Aziz R, Nahar N. Serum total protein and albumin levels in different grades of protein energy malnutrition. Journal of Bangladesh Society of Physiologist. 2009;**3**:58-60. DOI: 10.3329/jbsp.v3i0.1799

[28] Rosenbloom M et al. Vitamin toxicity. Medscape website. 2017

[29] Vitamin and Mineral Supplement Fact Sheets. Bethesda, MD: Office of Dietary Supplements, US National Institutes of Health; 2016 [Accessed: 19 December 2016]

[30] Zoroddu MA, Aashet J, Crisponi G, Medici S, Peana M, Nurchi VM. The essential metals for humans: A brief overview. Journal of Inorganic Biochemistry. 2019;**195**:120-129. DOI: 10.1016/j.jinorgbio.2019.03.013

[31] Minerals. MedlinePlus, National Library of Medicine, US National Institutes of Health; 2016 [Accessed: 24 December 2016]

[32] Minerals. Corvallis, OR: Micronutrient Information Center, Linus Pauling Institute, Oregon State University; 2016

[33] Richard R, Michael S. Wilson Disease. Seminars in Liver Disease. 2011;**31**(3):245-259

[34] Berdanier CD, Dwyer JT, Heber D. Handbook of Nutrition and Food. 3rd ed. CRC Press; 2016. pp. 211-224. ISBN: 978-1-4665-0572-8. [Accessed: 3 July 2016]

[35] Office of Dietary Supplements. Dietary Supplement Fact Sheet: Multivitamin/mineral Supplements. National Institutes of Health; 2019. Available from: http://ods.od.nih.gov/factsheets/MVMS-HealthProfessional/. Updated

[36] Bhalla K, Ennis DM, Ennis ED. Hypercalcemia caused by iatrogenic hypervitaminosis A. Journal of the American Dietetic Association. 2005;**105**(1):119-121

[37] Klein EA, Thompson IM Jr, Tangen CM, Crowley JJ, Lucia MS, Goodman PJ, et al. Vitamin E and the risk of prostate cancer: The selenium and vitamin E cancer prevention trial (SELECT). JAMA. 2011;**306**(14):1549-1556

[38] Corrigan JJ Jr, Marcus FI. Coagulopathy associated with vitamin E ingestion. JAMA. 1974;**230**(9):1300-1301

[39] Diplock AT. Safety of antioxidant vitamins and beta-carotene. American Journal of Clinical Nutrition. 1995;**62**(6 Suppl):1510S-1516S

[40] Office of Dietary Supplements. Dietary Supplement Fact Sheet: Vitamin B6. National Institutes of Health; 2011. Available from: http://ods.od.nih.gov/factsheets/VitaminB6-HealthProfessional/

[41] Fritz H, Flower G, Weeks L, Cooley K, Callachan M, McGowan J, et al. Intravenous vitamin C and cancer: A systematic review. Integrative Cancer Therapies. 2014;**13**(4):280-300

[42] Nordqvist C. Iron overload disorder: All you need to know. In: Medical News Today. 2017 Available from: https://www.medicalnewstoday.com/articles/166455.php

[43] Lederer E. Hypokalaemia. Medscape. 2018

[44] Simon EE. Hyponatremia. Medscape.

[45] Lukitsch I. 2018. Hypernatremia. Medscape.

[46] Desai J. Hypochloremic alkalosis. Medscape. 2018

[47] Luo EK. All you need to know about hyperchloremia. 2017

[48] Thomas EG. Hypercalcemia in Emergency Medicine. Medscape. 2018

[49] Suneja M. Hypocalcaemia. Medscape. 2019

[50] Silva Avila D, Luiz Puntel R, Aschner M. Chapter 7. Manganese in Health and Disease. In: Astrid S, Helmut S, RKO S, editors. Interrelations between Essential Metal Ions and Human Diseases. Metal Ions in Life Sciences. Vol. 13. Springer; 2013. pp. 199-227. DOI: 10.1007/978-94-007-7500-8_7

[51] Couper J. Sur les effets du peroxide de manganèse. Journal de Chimie Médicale, de Pharmacie et de Toxicologie. 1837;**3**:223-225

[52] Roth JA. Homeostatic and toxic mechanisms regulating manganese uptake, retention, and elimination. Biological Research. 2006;**39**(1):45-57. DOI: 10.4067/S0716-97602006000100006

[53] Freund H, Atamian S, Fischer JE. Chromium deficiency during total parenteral nutrition. JAMA. 1979;**241**(5):496-498. DOI: 10.1001/jama.1979.03290310036012

[54] Chromium. In: Dietary Reference Intakes for Vitamin A, Vitamin K, Arsenic, Boron, Chromium, Chromium, Iodine, Iron, Manganese, Molybdenum, Nickel, Silicon, Vanadium, and Chromium. National Academy Press; 2001. pp. 197-223

[55] Megan Ware RDN LD. Chromium: Health benefits, sources, and potential risks. Medical News Today. 2017. Available from: https://www.medicalnewstoday.com/articles/288177.php

[56] Selenium. Archives of Internal Medicine. 2010;**170**(3):256-261. DOI: 10.1001/archinternmed.2009.495

[57] Selenium. WebMD LLC; 2005–2019

[58] Health Encyclopedia. Rochester, NY: University of Rochester Medical Center; 2019

[59] Cobalt Poisoning. Mount Sinai: Icahn School of Medicine; 2019

[60] Lazzerini M, Ronfani L. Oral zinc for treating diarrhea in children. Cochrane Database Systematic Reviews. 2008:CD005436

[61] Scrimgeour AG, Lukaski HC. Zinc and diarrheal disease: Current status and future perspectives. Current Opinion in Clinical Nutrition and Metabolic Care. 2008;**11**(6):711-717

[62] Manary MJ. Local production and provision of ready-to-use therapeutic food (RUTF) spread for the treatment of severe childhood malnutrition. Food and Nutrition Bulletin. 2006;**27**(3 Suppl):S83-S89. DOI: 10.1177/15648265060273S305

[63] Zeng L, Dibley MJ, Cheng Y, et al. Impact of micronutrient supplementation during pregnancy on birth weight, duration of gestation, and perinatal mortality in rural western China: Double blind cluster randomized controlled trial. BMJ. 2008;7(337):a2001

[64] Roberfroid D, Huybregts L, Lanou H, et al. Effects of maternal multiple micronutrient supplementation on fetal growth: A double-blind randomized controlled trial in rural Burkina Faso. American Journal of Clinical Nutrition. 2008;**88**(5):1330-1340

[65] Kipsang JK et al. Pellagra in isoniazid preventive and antiretroviral therapy. In: IDCases 17. Elsevier Ltd; 2019. pp. 2214-2509. DOI: 10.1016/j.idcr.2019.e00550 This is an open access article under the CC BY-NC-ND license http://creativecommons.org/licenses/by-nc-nd/4.0/

[66] Guzmán-de-Peña D. The destruction of aflatoxins in rn by "nixtamalización". In: Rai M, Varma A, editors. Mycotoxins in Food, Feed and Bioweapons. Berlin, Heidelberg: Springer-Verlag; 2010. pp. 39-49. DOI: 10.1007/978-3-642-00725-5_3. ISBN: 978-3-642-00724-8. [Accessed: 12 April 2019]

[67] Pasquale F, Elliot MB, Jock RA. Encyclopedia of Food Security and Sustainability. Amsterdam: Elsevier; 2019

[68] Latham MC. Human Nutrition in the Developing World. Food & Agriculture Organization; 1997. p. 183 ISBN : 9789251038185

[69] Rucker RB, Zempleni J, Suttie JW, McCormick DB. Handbook of Vitamins. 4th ed. CRC Press; 2010. p. 192 ISBN: 978-1-4200-0580-6

[70] Wacher C. Nixtamalization, a Mesoamerican technology to process maize at small-scale with great potential for improving the nutritional quality of maize based foods. 2003. [Accessed: 5 March 2018]

[71] De-Regil LM, Suchdev PS, Vist GE, Walleser S, Peña-Rosas JP. Home fortification of foods with multiple micronutrient powders for health and nutrition in children under two years of age. Cochrane Database Systematic Reviews. 2011, 2011;**9**:CD008959. DOI: 10.1002/14651858.CD008959.pub2

[72] Piwoz E, Sundberg S, Rooke J. Promoting healthy growth: What are the priorities for research and action? Advances in Nutrition (Bethesda, Md.). 2012;**3**:234-241

[73] World Health Organization. Updates on the Management of Severe Acute Malnutrition in Infants and Children. [Guideline]. 2018. Available from: http://apps.who.int/iris/bitstream/

handle/10665/95584/9789241506328_eng.pdf?sequence=1

[74] Management of Severe Malnutrition: A Manual for Physicians and Other Senior Health Workers. World Health Organization. 1999. [Accessed: 11 February 2011]

[75] World Health Organization. Management of Severe Malnutrition: A Manual for Physicians and Other Senior Health Workers. 1999. Retrieved 11 February 2011

[76] Morrison SR. Plumpy'Nut: The lifesaver that costs... well, peanuts. The Independent. 2013. [Accessed: 14 March 2017]

Section 2

Malnutrition and Global Determinats

Chapter 5

Wernicke Encephalopathy in Elderly Related to Severe Malnutrition

Francisco Javier Ros Forteza

Abstract

Wernicke encephalopathy (WE) is the main neurologic complication of thiamine deficiency. Thiamine is a cofactor for several key enzymes important in energy metabolism. WE is a little-recognised and underdiagnosed condition, and the prevalence in the elderly is unknown. The classic triad of WE includes encephalopathy, oculomotor dysfunction, and gait ataxia. Diagnosis is clinical, and early treatment with thiamine is fundamental in preventing coma and death. In the cases reported in the literature, the cause of WE was fasting or malnutrition in 10.2% of cases. WE may in some cases constitute a public health problem. Being the prevalence unknown, we alert clinicians to keep severe malnutrition in elderly as a form of precipitation of WE. We review the cases published in the literature.

Keywords: Wernicke encephalopathy, elderly, severe malnutrition, underdiagnosed condition, thiamine deficiency

1. Introduction

Wernicke encephalopathy (WE) is the main neurologic complication of thiamine deficiency. Thiamine is a cofactor for several key enzymes important in energy metabolism [1]. Although the chronic alcoholism is recognised as the most common cause of WE, malnutrition has also been less documented [2] generating deprivation of other micronutrients (including in addition to albumin; thiamine; riboflavin; pyridoxine; vitamins B12, E and D; niacin; folate; ferritin; calcium; and magnesium mainly). WE is an acute syndrome characterised by mental confusion, ophthalmoplegia, and gait ataxia (classic triad), but they are not always present which likely leads to under-diagnosis [3]. In chronic alcohol abusers, they have also been used the following four Caine criteria: dietary deficiency, oculomotor abnormalities, cerebellar dysfunction, and either altered mental status or mild memory impairment. Two of the four criteria are sufficient for the diagnosis [4]. Structural diseases of the medial thalamus, hippocampus, or the inferior medial region of the temporal lobe should also be considered due to the similar neuroanatomical involvement to WE. Diagnosis is clinical, and early treatment is fundamental in preventing coma and death. Imaging studies can be helpful but should not delay treatment.

2. Malnutrition among the elderly

Nutrition is a significant determinant of health. Undernutrition presenting as malnutrition is a serious health concern for frail elderly people with many health problems [5].

2.1 Diagnosis of malnutrition

The following criteria for the diagnosis of malnutrition have been recommended in a consensus statement from the Academy of Nutrition and Dietetics (Academy) and the American Society for Parenteral and enteral Nutrition (ASPEN) [6].

Two or more of the following six characteristics:

- Insufficient energy intake.
- Weight loss (according to Zawada, 1996) is considered to be clinically significant with the following parameters: >2% decrease of baseline body weight in 1 month; >5% decrease in 3 months, or > 10% in 6 months.
- Loss of muscle mass.
- Loss of subcutaneous fat.
- Localised or generalised fluid accumulation that may mask weight loss.
- Diminished functional status as measured by handgrip strength.

2.2 Population at risk

The people most at risk are the frail elderly and with few or no social and environmental support [5]. These patients may have signs of nutritional deficiency living institutionalised or being hospitalised that can go unnoticed. They are clinical conditions that increase the use of thiamine and may precipitate WE in patients with marginal thiamine reserves such as poor dietary intake, unbalanced nutrition, prolonged intravenous feeding, terminal cancer, and gastrointestinal surgery.

2.3 Epidemiology of malnutrition

The epidemiology of malnutrition depends on the definition used, although in most studies it refers to the undernutrition concerning weight loss and deficiency of nutritional components. Housebound and institutionalised elderly people have most frequently been shown to be deficient in vitamins A, C, D, B complex, folic acid, and B_{12} as well as calcium, iron, and zinc [5].

Nutritional deficiencies are ranked in the top 20 leading worldwide disease and disability burden in 2016, according to the Institute of Health Metrics Evaluation [7].

The prevalence of malnutrition in hospitalised adults has been extensively reported in the international literature and varies between 13 and 78% among acute-care patients [8]. The vulnerability in data may be due to terminology used, the diagnostic criteria, and variations in communities.

2.4 Aetiology of malnutrition

In examining the aetiology of malnutrition, we must consider risk factors that could cause the condition or exacerbate the underlying cause. Morley [9] has developed a mnemonic *meals-on-wheels* for identifying potentially treatable causes of malnutrition (adapted from Morley):

Medications; emotional problems (depression); anorexia nervosa (tardive) and abnormal attitudes to food; late-life paranoia; swallowing problems; oral problems; no money (especially those on fixed incomes); wandering and other dementia-related behaviours; hyperthyroidism; hyperparathyroidism; entry problems (malabsorption); eating problems (physical and cognitive); low-salt, low-cholesterol diets; and shopping (food availability).

2.5 Consequences of malnutrition

We know that malnutrition can lead to a weak immune system, which increases the risk of infections, a muscle weakness, a decreased bone mass, a higher risk of hospitalisation, and an increased risk of death.

According to Saunders J et al., 2011, the most relevant consequences of malnutrition on health include increased risk of infections, functional decline, delayed wound healing, cognitive decline, impaired respiratory function, muscle weakness and depression, delayed recovery from acute illness, and increased mortality [10].

2.6 Neurological disorders associated with malnutrition

- Neurological disorders caused by nutrient deficiency (**Table 1**)
- Potentially toxic food compounds that may contribute to neurological disorders (**Table 2**)

3. Thiamine deficiency in elderly people

Thiamine (vitamin B1), as thiamine pyrophosphate (TPP), is an essential coenzyme in several important energy yielding reactions, including the transketolase reaction in the pentose phosphate pathway.

We cognize that the recommended daily allowance for an adult is 1.1 mg/dl and the current UK recommended nutrient intake for elderly people is 0.4 mg of thiamine per 1000 kcal [11]. Also, there is evidence that subclinical thiamine deficiency may contribute to anorexia in the elderly [12].

The reported prevalence in the UK ranges from 8 to 31% for elderly people living at home and from 23 to 40% for those in nursing homes [13]. Biochemical thiamine deficiency has also been reported in 48% of patients admitted to an acute geriatric unit [13].

3.1 Thiamine deficiency in developed countries

Alcoholism is the most common cause of thiamine depletion in developed countries. Alcohol interferes with the active intestinal transport of vitamin B1. In chronic hepatopathy, the ability to store thiamine and transform it into its active form is diminished. The affinity of transketolase for thiamine pyrophosphate may be genetically decreased in some people, which predispose them to WE. A diet rich in carbohydrates or the administration of serum glucose in a patient with masked deficiency of vitamin B1 precipitates or aggravates EW, even to death. Thiamine reserves do not exceed 3 weeks, so it is not difficult to present a deficit in acute situations (e.g. post-surgery status, prolonged hospitalisation in intensive care unit, hunger strikes, etc.) [14].

Nutrient	RDA*	Neurological disorder when deficient
Macronutrients		
Total energy	2200 (kcal)	In childhood: long-term mental deficit
Vitamins		
Vitamin A	600 μg	Night-blindness
Vitamin B1 (thiamine)	1.1 mg	Beriberi, polyneuropathy, Wernicke encephalopathy, Korsakoff syndrome
Vitamin B3 (niacin)	15 mg NE	Pellagra including dementia and depression. Neuropsychiatric disorders
Vitamin B6 (pyridoxine)	1.6 mg	Polyneuropathy. neuropsychiatric disorders including seizures, migraine, chronic pain, and depression
Vitamin B12 (cobalamin)	2.0 μg	Progressive myelopathy with sensory disturbances in the legs. Ataxia. Dementia. Neuropsychiatric disorders
Vitamin D3 (cholecalciferol)	5 μg	Myopathy
Vitamin E (alpha-tocopherol)	10 mg	Ataxia, myopathy, retinopathy/ophthalmoplegia
Folate	180 μg	Neural tube defects (myelomeningocele) of the fetus, cognitive dysfunction in children and elderly. Neuropsychiatric disorders. Increased vascular risk (in hyper-homocysteine)
Minerals		
Iodine	150 μg	Iodine deficiency disorders: Cretinism (severe mental retardation, growth retardation, deaf-mutism, and physical disability). Decrease in IQ and lower school performance
Iron	15 mg	Delayed mental development in children
Zinc	12 mg	Delayed motor development in children, behavioural abnormalities, and depression. Visual disturbances
Selenium	55 mg	Adverse mood states, myopathy
Magnesium	400 mg	Behavioural, sleep, and memory abnormalities. Tremor and weakness. Depression. Seizures
Manganeso	2 mg	Behavioural and memory abnormalities. Seizures

**Recommended daily allowance for an adult.*
Source: Diop et al. [15] (completed by Ros Forteza).

Table 1.
Neurological disorders caused by nutrient deficiency.

3.2 Wernicke encephalopathy

For WE and Korsakoff syndrome (KS), there are the acute phase and the residual state, respectively, of the same pathological process. Both are the result of thiamine deficiency.

It can occur at any age, and although it is more frequent in men, women are more susceptible [1].

Thiamine has an important role in catabolism of carbohydrates and neurotransmitter formation. Its utilisation depends on the individual's metabolic rate, increasing with a higher energy requirement [16].

In the gastrointestinal tract, this nutrient is actively absorbed at the duodenum level and then transported through the blood–brain barrier by passive and active processes [17].

Food compound	Potential neurological disorder when ingested
Alcohol	Fetal alcohol syndrome, retarded mental development in childhood, delirium, cerebral atrophy, dementia, Wernicke encephalopathy, Korsakoff syndrome, visual problems (amblyopia), ataxia, peripheral neuropathy, myopathy, epilepsy
Lathyrus sativus	Spastic paraparesis (lathyrism)
Cyanogenic glucosides from insufficiently processed cassava roots	Konzo (tropic ataxic neuropathy)

Source: Diop et al. [15] (completed by Ros Forteza).

Table 2.
Potentially toxic food compounds that may contribute to neurological disorders.

In its biologically active form (thiamine pyrophosphate), it is an essential coenzyme for various enzymes of catabolism of glucose-6-phosphate, such as transketolase, pyruvate dehydrogenase, and α-ketoglutarate dehydrogenase [17, 18]. The first enzyme participates in the pentose-phosphate pathway, and its catalytic activity results in reduced ribose-5-phosphate and nicotinamide adenosine dinucleotide (NADPH) molecules. Both are crucial in the synthesis of various other compounds (e.g. nucleic acids and glutathione), and any cell requires optimal levels of these enzymes. The other two enzymes catalyse glycolysis and Krebs cycle reactions, respectively. These metabolic pathways result in the formation of adenosine triphosphate (ATP) molecules, vital in providing energy for cell metabolism. Low levels of mentioned enzymes lead to lower energy synthesis and cell death [18].

As thiamine reserves (30–50 mg) do not exceed 3 weeks, it is not difficult for a deficit to occur in acute situations. In some cases, low levels of magnesium, an essential cofactor of thiamine into its active diphosphate and triphosphate forms, have been implicated with thiamine deficiency in WE [19].

Only a subset of thiamine-deficient alcohol abusers develop WE. Investigators have found that in alcohol abusers with WE, the thiamine-dependent enzyme transketolase has an altered affinity for thiamine. Variants in the high affinity thiamine transporter gene have also been implicated [20].

The classic triad of WE includes encephalopathy, oculomotor dysfunction, and gait ataxia; these were recognised in only one-third of patients. The encephalopathy is characterised by profound disorientation, indifference, and inattentiveness. The ocular signs consist of nystagmus that is both horizontal and vertical and mainly evoked by gaze; this is the most common feature, weakness, or paralysis of the lateral rectus muscles and weakness or paralysis of conjugate gaze. Usually there is some combination of these abnormalities, according to Adams and Victor's, 2014. Ataxia primarily involves stance and gait and is likely due to a combination of polyneuropathy, cerebellar involvement, and vestibular dysfunction [1].

In one study of 106 autopsied alcohol abusers, the Caine criteria (two of four being enough: dietary deficiency, oculomotor abnormalities, cerebellar dysfunction, either altered mental status or mild memory impairment) increased the diagnostic sensitivity for WE from 22% using the classic triad to 85% [4].

Other signs in patients with WE may also be present as vestibular dysfunction without hearing loss; the presence of spontaneous nystagmus with absent caloric responses appears to be a relatively specific finding in WE [21]. Additionally, peripheral neuropathy, hypothermia, and cardiovascular signs and symptoms such as tachycardia, exertional dyspnoea, elevated cardiac output, and EKG abnormalities can be detected [1]. These reverse with thiamine administration.

Imaging studies should not delay treatment, especially a MRI. However, diagnostic imaging can be helpful by providing evidence of WE in many patients and may rule out alternative diagnoses [20].

Typical findings include lesions surrounding the aqueduct and third ventricle and within the medial thalamus, dorsal medulla, tectal plate, and mammillary bodies. Lesions may also be seen in atypical areas such as the cerebellum, cranial nerve nuclei, dentate nuclei, caudate, red nuclei, splenium, and cerebral cortex. Abnormal T2 signal disappears within as little as 48 h after treatment with thiamine [20]. Mammillary body atrophy is a relatively specific abnormality in patients with chronic lesions of WE [22] and can be detected within 1 week of the onset of WE [23].

There are no laboratory studies that are diagnostic of WE. WE is primarily a clinical diagnosis. WE should be considered in the differential diagnosis of all patients presenting with acute delirium or acute ataxia [20]. Also, structural diseases in the medial thalami, hippocampi, or inferior medial temporal lobes should be considered because of the neuroanatomic overlap with WE. These include top-of-the-basilar stroke, hypoxic–ischemic encephalopathy after cardiac arrest, herpes simplex encephalitis, and third ventricular tumours [24, 25].

The diagnosis of WE is difficult to confirm and, when untreated, most patients progress to coma and death. Therefore, diagnostic testing (measurement of biochemical thiamine deficiency [13]) should not delay treatment, which should immediately follow the consideration of the diagnosis [20].

Patients with suspected WE require immediate parenteral administration of thiamine. A recommended regimen is 500 mg of thiamine intravenously, infused over 30 min, 3 times daily for two consecutive days and 250 mg intravenously or intramuscularly once daily for an additional 5 days, in combination with other B vitamins. There are no randomised studies to support a particular dosing regimen. Administration of glucose without thiamine can precipitate or worsen WE; thus, thiamine should be administered before glucose. Subsequently daily 100 mg oral thiamine should be continued until patients are no longer considered at risk [20].

The disappearance of nystagmus and an improvement in ophthalmoparesis within hours or a day of the administration of thiamine confirms the diagnosis. Ataxia recovery begins during the second week, and confusion declines over days and weeks according to Adams and Victor, 2014. MRI resolves with clinical improvement. Only a minority of such patients (fewer than 20% in Victor's series) recover entirely.

4. Wernicke encephalopathy in elderly related to severe malnutrition

4.1 Justification and literature

The absence of a nutritional assessment method that can be considered a "gold standard" makes it very difficult to task. Also unfortunately there is no data in the medical records about nutritional evaluation nor in publications outside the field of nutrition, and healthcare professionals receive little education on nutrition. For these reasons all healthcare professionals should be involved and not just the nutritionist in this public health problem.

There are few cases published in the literature of WE in elderly related to malnutrition [26–32].

Magalhães Scoralick et al. describe a case of a 63-year-old man with grade IV chagasic mega oesophagus who developed WE. There was no past of alcohol, and the patient had not received nutritional therapy, and he was not taking a vitamin supplement. The deficiency of vitamins B1 and B6 was found. The patient recovered from the acute symptoms; however 3 months after his admission, he died [26].

Another case of WE was due to dual deficiency of both thiamine (vitamin B1) and niacin (vitamin A PP) in an 80-year-old woman regular consumer of alcohol with severe malnutrition; vitamin D and B6 deficits were also found [27].

Differently, a case of autopsy-proven acute nonalcoholic thiamine-deficient encephalopathy without medical treatment antemortem. The patient was found dead in his room; he was a 62-year-old man and had BMI 11.7, and vitamin B1 and B12 deficits were detected [28].

On the other hand, other authors report a WE and pellagra in an alcoholic and malnourished patient. He was a 61-year-old man and had a vitamin deficiency of B1 and niacin. Thiamine and nicotinic acid were administered. Finally, the patient was transferred to a rehabilitation facility, where he gained the support of an alcohol abstinence education programme [29].

Also the case of a 65-year-old female, nonalcoholic with a 43-Kg weight loss (25% of baseline weight) over several weeks. On admission, she received a continuous intravenous glucose infusion, and 4 days later she developed symptoms suggestive of WE. A brain MRI demonstrated signal change in the medial thalami and mammillary bodies. The patient received intravenous thiamine therapy and was discharged on oral thiamine with clinical improvement [30].

We highlight a series of five elderly patients whose brain showed typical features of WE at the autopsy. All five were females with a mean age of 67 +/− years-old. One case was alcoholic, but the other four were nonalcoholics and developed the disease after prolonged malnutrition. WE was diagnosed clinically only in one case [31].

4.2 Special case report

We present the case [32] of an 81-year-old autonomous woman with 10 years of schooling and body mass index (BMI) previously of 23.2. There was no history of tobacco and alcohol use. Her medical history included hypertension, acute biliary pancreatitis, and hiatal hernia diagnosed 18 years previously. Her surgical history incorporated cholecystectomy and anti-reflux surgery 15 years previously. She was being treated with candesartan, pantoprazole, domperidone, ursodeoxycholic acid, mirtazapine, mexazolam, and brotizolam. Two to three weeks after an influenza episode, she developed anorexia, dehydration, mental confusion, altered sleep–wake cycle, and visual and gait impairment..

On physical examination, the patient showed somnolence, but easily aroused, disorientation in time but not space, incoherent speech, strabismus, persistent horizontal-rotary nystagmus, dysphagia for liquids, and hypotonia. A second head CT scan at 24 h revealed a suspected lacunar stroke of the right tectal plate (**Figure 1A**), requiring examination with brain MRI. A transthoracic echocardiography and lumbar puncture had normal results.

She started treatment with thiamine at high doses (500 mg IV every 8 h for 2 days, 500 mg IV every 24 h for 5 days), then at 100 mg IV every 8 h during the remaining days of hospitalisation, combined with a multivitamin solution [vitamins A, B, H (biotin), and F] and protein-calorie supplementation. We observed a significant clinical improvement, with decreased nystagmus, improved verbal expression, and corrected sleep pattern. A brain MRI (**Figure 1B-G**) performed at day 5 of admission revealed diffuse hyperintensity of the tectum, periaqueductal region, medial thalami, mammillary bodies, and structures adjacent to the diencephalon and cortical convexity with brain atrophy, which were indicative of WE.

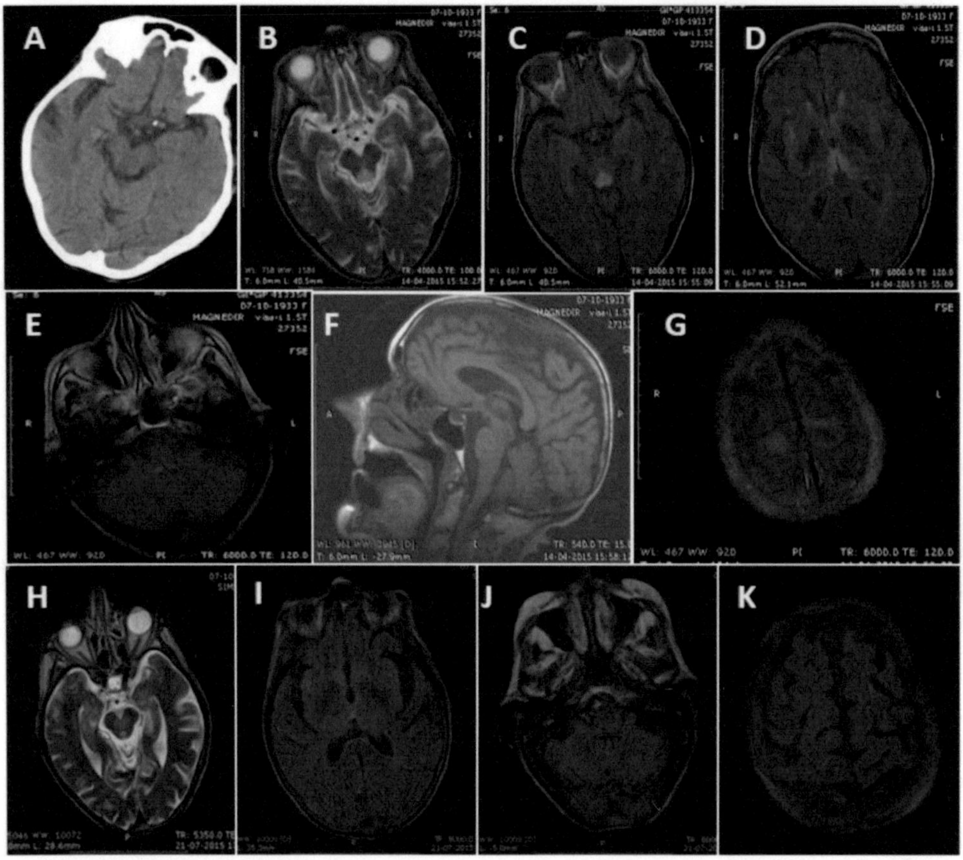

Figure 1.
Published with permission of the editor. Source: Ros Forteza et al. [32]. Baseline findings: *(A) head CT at 24 h: Hypodensity in the right tectal plate. (B) Axial T2-weighted MRI sequence. (C) Axial FLAIR MRI sequence: Lesion to the midbrain periaqueductal region. (D) Axial FLAIR MRI sequence: Bilateral thalamic lesions. (E) Axial FLAIR MRI sequence: Tectal lesion. (F) Sagittal T1-weighted MRI sequence: no alterations. (G) Axial FLAIR MRI sequence: Lesion to the superior frontal cortex and pia mater.* Findings at resolution: *(H) axial T2-weighted MRI sequence: Regressing periaqueductal lesion. (I) Axial FLAIR MRI sequence: no thalamic lesion. (J) Axial FLAIR MRI sequence: no bulbar lesion. (K) Axial FLAIR MRI sequence: no lesion to the cortex or pia mater.*

At day 6 of admission, the patient was awake, with no spontaneous verbal response, exotropia of the right eye, and mild horizontal-rotatory nystagmus. Other tests were apparently normal. The BMI was 15.6.

Extensive work-up revealed a decrease in haemoglobin, vitamin B1 (27 ng/mL), vitamin B12, vitamin D, magnesium, sodium, and albumin. Intrinsic factor antibody test and serological test for syphilis yielded negative results.

Thiamine was maintained at 100 mg IV every 8 h; pantoprazole was withdrawn, and ranitidine started at 150 mg at night. The patient also started treatment with oral vitamin B12 at 5 mg/day, cholecalciferol 667 IU/day, magnesium 10 mL/12 h, calcium carbonate 500 mg/12 h, and 0.9% saline solution. During the first 2 weeks of admission, her speech improved, and she was able to produce sentences; nystagmus manifested only at extreme lateral gaze. Ataxic gait was later identified, and she started rehabilitation.

At 1 month of admission, an awake EEG revealed slow background activity, suggesting diffuse brain dysfunction (grades 2–3). From the second month of treatment, our patient presented good general appearance, fluent and coherent speech, and an MMSE score of 23. The patient participated in craft activities and regular rehabilitation sessions.

At 3 months of admission, a brain MRI scan demonstrated complete remission of the brain lesions (**Figure 1H–K**).

The neuropsychological evaluation showed that autobiographical memory was preserved. We were able to apply only three subtests of the Wechsler Adult Intelligence Scale (WAIS-III): matrix reasoning, similarities, and digit span; results were higher level, average level, and average level, respectively. No areas of deficit were identified.

The age of our patient was atypical with clinical presentation of the classic triad. In this case, WE was caused by severe malnutrition [2]. The patient lost 33% of her body weight, with a BMI of 15.6 [BMI below 16 corresponds to grade 3/severe thinness according to the WHO classifications (1995, 2000)]. Protein-calorie deficiency is not always present; in a review of 625 cases reported in the literature, the cause of WE was fasting or malnutrition in 10.2% of cases [33].

Brain MRI showed typical findings of WE, although this test is more sensitive for detecting WE lesions in non-alcoholic than in alcoholic patients [34]; clinical recovery was excellent with vitamin supplementation.

Regarding the pathophysiology of these symptoms, thiamine reserves were depleted in 2–3 weeks due to caloric restriction. In the event of thiamine depletion, the function of the thiamine-dependent enzyme systems deteriorates, and blood thiamine levels decrease. This damage occurs 4 days after the onset of thiamine deficiency and eventually progresses to programmed cell death. At 14 days, brain lesions develop [2]. It is probable that some subjects with genetically reduced transketolase activity require higher levels of thiamine and therefore present a higher risk of WE in situations of increased demand or lower absorption [34].

Additionally, the low level of magnesium (a thiamine cofactor) also contributed to the genesis of this clinical picture. Many cases of WE may also have magnesium (Mg) depletion, and it is known that in elderly people, Mg intake may be suboptimum. If a depletion of Mg reserve impedes the phosphorylation of thiamine, Mg depletion could have an effect on other enzymes hose activities depending on Mg [35]. Other vitamin deficiencies were vitamin B12 and vitamin D. It is recognised that long-term use of pantoprazole suppresses gastric acid production, which may lead to vitamin B12 malabsorption [36].

This case is special because being the clinical picture of several weeks of evolution, the first diagnostic hypothesis was vertebrobasilar stroke. WE was diagnosed in a context of severe malnutrition little evident in a nonalcoholic patient, despite symptoms (complete classic triad present) and neuroimaging findings being more typical (except alterations of cerebral cortex) of an alcoholic patient [34]. There was also no atrophy of the mammillary bodies, a very specific pathological finding in chronic EW and KS and present in up to 80% of alcoholic patients with a history of EW [37–39].

We propose that WE should be considered in elderly patients with mental status changes of unknown cause and risk for thiamine deficiency, even in nonalcoholic patients. Infusion of thiamine should be started immediately when the disorder is suspected, even in the absence of typical symptoms. With this case, we aim to raise awareness of the need to identify this preventable, treatable, and high-mortality disease.

4.3 Future perspectives

Nowadays, despite the caloric density, the diet is often of poor nutrition quality and does not meet recommended dietary guidelines for micronutrient intake, making this an at-risk population for micronutrient malnutrition [40].

On the other hand, genetic factors may be involved in thiamine deficiency, i.e. pathogenic gene mutations in key regulators of the thiamine pathway, including thiamine pyrophosphokinase 1 (TPK1), thiamine diphosphate kinase (TDPK), thiamine triphosphatase (THTPA), and thiamine transporters (SLC25A19, SLC19A2/THTR1, and SLC19A3/THTR2) [40]. More recently, it has been defended that the organic cation transporter 1 (OCT1) plays a role as a hepatic thiamine transporter [41].

In addition, oxidative stress also is involved in this disease. In the near future, supplemental antioxidants will be incorporated for the prevention and treatment of the EW.

5. Conclusion

WE in elderly related to severe malnutrition is a little-recognised and underdiagnosed condition. Beyond an anamnesis of suspicion and a timely neurological semiology, nutrition education is necessary, and this information must be explicit in the clinical records. Parenteral thiamine should be given to all at-risk subjects admitted to the emergency room, and in every patient with WE, other nutritional deficiencies must be searched. It is necessary that a collaborative network of researchers in the field of malnutrition in older patients and clinicians should raise awareness of the need to identify this preventable, treatable, and high-mortality disease.

Conflict of interest

There is no conflict of interest.

Author details

Francisco Javier Ros Forteza[1,2]

1 Neurology Service, Local Health Unit of Guarda, E.P.E., Guarda, Portugal

2 Department of Medical Sciences, Faculty of Health Sciences, University of Beira Interior, Covilhã, Portugal

*Address all correspondence to: javierros40@hotmail.com

References

[1] Victor M, Adams RA, Collins GH. The Wernicke-Korsakoff Syndrome and Related Disorders Due to Alcoholism and Malnutrition. Philadelphia: FA Davis; 1989

[2] Hutcheon DA. Malnutrition-induced Wernicke's encephalopathy following a water-only fasting diet. Nutrition in Clinical Practice. 2015;**30**:92-99

[3] Harper CG, Giles M, Finlay-Jones R. Clinical signs in the Wernicke-Korsakoff complex: A retrospective analysis of 131 cases diagnosed at necropsy. Journal of Neurology, Neurosurgery, and Psychiatry. 1986;**49**:341-345

[4] Caine D, Halliday GM, Kril JJ, Harper CG. Operational criteria for the classification of chronic alcoholics: Identification of Wernicke's encephalopathy. Journal of Neurology, Neurosurgery, and Psychiatry. 1997;**62**:51

[5] Rauscher C. Canadian Family Physian. Malnutrition among the Elderly. 1993;**39**:1395-1403

[6] White JV, Guenter P, Jensen G, et al. Consensu statement: Academy of nutrition ans dietetics and American Society for Parenteral and Enteral Nutrition: Characteristics recommended for the identification and documentation of adult malnutrition (undernutrition). Journal of Parenteral and Enteral Nutrition. 2012;**36**:275

[7] Ritchie H, Roser M. Micronutrient Deficiency. 2018. Published online at OurWorldInData.org. Retrieved from: https://ourworldindata.org/micronutrient-deficiency

[8] van Tonder E, Gardner L, Cressey S, Tydeman-Edwards R, Gerber K. Adult malnutrition: Prevalence and use of nutrition-related quality indicators in south African public-sector hospitals. South African Journal of Clinical Nutrition. 2017;**32**(1):1-7

[9] Bernard M, Rombeau J. Nutritional support for the elderly patient. In: Young E, editor. Nutrition, Ageing and Health. New York: Alan R. Liss Inc; 1986. pp. 229-258

[10] Saunders J, Smith T, Stroud M. Malnutrition and undernutrition. Medicine. 2011;**39**:45-50

[11] Department of Health and Social Security. Dietary Reference Values for Food Energy and Nutrients for the United Kingdom. Report on Health and Social Subjects, no. 41. London: HMSO; 1991

[12] Smidt LJ, Cremin FM, Grivetti LE, Clifford AJ. Influence of thiamin supplementation on the health and general well-being of an elderly Irish population with marginal thiamin deficiency. Journal of Gerontology. 1991;**46**:M16-M22

[13] O'Keeffe ST. Thiamine deficiency in elderly people. Age and Ageing. 2000;**29**:99-101

[14] Zarranz JJ, Pérez-Concha T. Enfermedades carenciales. In: Zarranz JJ, editor. Neurologia. 3nd ed. Madrid: Elsevier Science; 2003. pp. 879-886

[15] Diop AG, Millogo A, Obot I, Thiam I, Tylleskar T. Neurological disorders associated with malnutrition. In: Aarli JA, Avanzini G, Bertolote JM, de Boer H, Breivik H, Dua T, et al., editors. Neurological Disorders: Public Health Challenges. World Health Organization, Geneva. 2006. p. 111-126

[16] Tanphaichitr V. Thiamin. In: Shils ME, Olson JA, Shike M, Ross AC,

editors. Modern Nutrition in Health and Disease. 9th ed. Baltimore: Williams and Wilkins; 1999. pp. 381-389

[17] Thomson AD, Cook CCH, Touquet R, Henry JA. The Royal College of Physicians report on alcohol: Guidelines for managing Wernicke's encephalopathy in the accident and emergency department. Alcohol and Alcoholism. Supplement. 2002;**37**:513-521

[18] Martin PR, Singleton CK, Hiller-Sturmhöfel S. The role of thiamine deficiency in alcoholic brain disease. Alcohol Research & Health. 2003;**27**:134

[19] McLean J, Manchip S. Wernicke's encephalopathy induced by magnesium depletion. Lancet. 1999;**353**:1768

[20] So YT, Aminoff MJ, Wilterdink JL. Wernicke encephalopathy. UpToDate May 2019;1-18

[21] Goor C, Endtz LJ, Muller Kobold MJ. Electro-nystagmography for the diagnosis of vestibular dysfunction in the Wernicke-Korsakow syndrome. Clinical Neurology and Neurosurgery. 1975;**78**:112

[22] Charness ME. Intracranial voyeurism: Revealing the mammillary bodies in alcoholism. Alcoholism, Clinical and Experimental Research. 1999;**23**:1941

[23] Park SH, Kim M, Na DL, Jeon BS. Magnetic resonance reflects the pathological evolution of Wernicke encephalopathy. Journal of Neuroimaging. 2001;**11**:406

[24] Yoneoka Y, Takeda N, Inoue A, et al. Acute Korsakoff syndrome following mammillothalamic tract infarction. AJNR. American Journal of Neuroradiology. 2004;**25**:964

[25] Renou P, Ducreux D, Batouche F, Denier C. Pure and acute Korsakoff syndrome due to a bilateral anterior fornix infarction: A diffusion tensor tractography study. Archives of Neurology. 2008;**65**:1252

[26] Magalhães Scoralick F, Louzada LL, Toledo MA, Ruback M. Wernicke's encephalopathy as a complication of Chagas mega esophagus. Journal of Aging Research & Clinical Practice. 2012;**1**(2):178-180

[27] Chidlovskii E, Tahar A, Deschasse G, Couturier P. Wernicke's encephalopathy associated with pellagra encephalopathy: Rare and unusual complication in an elderly hospitalized for aspiration pneumonia. La Revue de médicine interne. 2012;**33**:453-456

[28] Hata Y, Takeuchi Y, Kinoshita K, Nishida N. An autopsy case of acute and nonalcoholic thiamine-deficient encephalopathy. European Neurology. 2014;**71**:230-232

[29] Terada N, Kinoshita K, Taguchi S, Tokuda Y. Wernicke encephalopathy and pellagra in an alcoholic and malnourished patient. BML Case Reports. 2015:Oct 21. DOI: 10.1136/bcr-2015-209412

[30] Nariai H, Mittelmann E, Farmakidis C, Zampolin RL, Robbins MS. Bithalamic dysfunction in Wernicke's encephalopathy. The Einstein Journal of Biology and Medicine. 2016;**31**:23-24

[31] Yokote K, Yamanouchi H, Mizutani T, Shimada H. Clinical characteristics of Wernicke's encephalopathy in the elderly. Nihon Ronen Igakkai Zasshi. 1992;**29**:35-40

[32] Ros Forteza FJ, Cabrera H, Bousende M. Malnutrition and Wernicke encephalopathy in the elderly. Neurología. 2018;**34**:543-546. DOI: 10.1016/j.nrleng.2018.11.005

[33] Galvin R, Brathen G, Ivashynka A, Hillbom M, Tanasescu R, Leone MA.

EFNS guidelines for diagnosis, therapy and prevention of Wernicke encephalopathy. European Journal of Neurology. 2010;**17**:1408-1418

[34] Gascón-Bayarri J, Campdelacreu J, García-Carreira MC, Estela J, Martínez-Yélamos S, Palasí A, et al. Encefalopatía de Wernicke en pacientes no alcohólicos: una serie de 8 casos. Neurología. 2011;**26**:540-547

[35] McLean J, Manchip S. Wernicke's encephalopathy induced by magnesium depletion. The Lancet. 1999;**353**:1768

[36] Lam JR, Schneider JL, Zhao W, Corley DA. Proton pump inhibitor and histamine 2 receptor antagonist use and vitamin B12 deficiency. Journal of the American Medical Association. 2013;**310**:2435-2442

[37] Skullerud K, Andersen SN, Lundevall J. Cerebral lesions and causes of death in male alcoholics. A forensic autopsy study. International Journal of Legal Medicine. 1991;**104**:209-213

[38] Charness ME. Intracranial voyeurism: Revealing the mammillary bodies in alcoholism. Alcoholism, Clinical and Experimental Research. 1999;**23**:1941

[39] Zuccoli G, Pipitone N. Neuroimaging findings in acute Wernicke's encephalopathy: Review of the literature. American Journal of Roentgenology. 2009;**192**:501-508

[40] Dhir S, Tarasenko M, Napoli E, Giulivi C. Neurological, psychiatric and biochemical aspects of thiamine deficiency in children and adults. Frontiers in Psychiatry. 2019;**10**:207. DOI: 10.3389/fpsyt.2019.00207

[41] Chen L, Yee SW, Giacomini KM. OCT1 in hepatic steatosis and thiamine disposition. Cell Cycle. 2015;**14**:283-284. DOI: 10.1080/15384101.2015.1006532

Chapter 6

Global Prevalence of Malnutrition: Evidence from Literature

Natisha Dukhi

Abstract

Malnutrition is a widespread problem, affecting the global population at some life stage. This public health epidemic targets everyone, but the most vulnerable groups are poverty-stricken people, young children, adolescents, older people, those who are with illness and have a compromised immune system, as well as lactating and pregnant women. Malnutrition includes both undernutrition (wasting, stunting, underweight, and mineral- and vitamin-related malnutrition) and overnutrition (overweight, obesity, and diet-related noncommunicable diseases). In combating malnutrition, healthcare costs increase, productivity is reduced, and economic growth is staggered, thus perpetuating the cycle of ill health and poverty. The best-targeted age for addressing malnutrition is the first 1000 days of life as this window period is ideal for intervention implementation and tracking for the improvement of child growth and development. There is an unprecedented opportunity to address the various forms of malnutrition, especially the 2016–2025 Decade of Action on Nutrition set by the United Nation. This aims to achieve the relevant targets of the Sustainable Development Goals that aim to end hunger and improve nutrition, as well as promote well-being and ensure healthy lives.

Keywords: malnutrition, children, wasting, stunting, obesity

1. Introduction

Malnutrition is a universal public health problem in both children and adults globally [1]. It is not only a public health concern but it is an impediment to global poverty eradication, productivity and economic growth. By eliminating malnutrition, it is estimated that 32% of the global disease burden would be removed [2]. As a widespread serious problem affecting children in developing countries, progress towards tackling the different forms of malnutrition remains relatively slow [3]. Malnutrition occurs due to an imbalance in the body, whereby the nutrients required by the body and the amount used by the body do not balance [1]. There are several forms of malnutrition and these include two broad categories namely undernutrition and over nutrition. Undernutrition manifests as wasting or low weight for height (acute malnutrition), stunting or low height for age (chronic malnutrition), underweight or low weight for age, and mineral and vitamin deficiencies or excessiveness. Over nutrition includes overweight, obesity and diet-related non-communicable diseases (NCDs) such as diabetes mellitus, heart disease, some forms of cancer and stroke [1]. Malnutrition is an important global issue currently, as it affects all people despite the geography, socio-economic status, sex and gender, overlapping households, communities and countries. Anyone can experience malnutrition but the most vulnerable groups affected are children, adolescents, women, as well as people who are immune-compromised, or facing the challenges of poverty [3].

According to the World Health Organization (WHO), 462 million adults are underweight, while 1.9 billion adults are overweight and/or obese. In children under 5 years of age, 155 million are stunted, 52 million are wasted, 17 million are severely wasted and 41 million are overweight and/or obese [1]. The manifestation of malnutrition is multifold, but the paths to addressing prevention are key and include exclusive breastfeeding for the first 2 years of life, diverse and nutritious foods during childhood, healthy environments, access to basic services such as water, hygiene, health and sanitation, as well as pregnant and lactating women having proper maternal nutrition before, during and after the respective phases (levels and trends) [3].

It is vital that malnutrition is addressed in children as malnutrition manifestations and symptoms begin to appear in the first 2 years of life [4]. Coinciding with the mental development and growth periods in children, protein energy malnutrition (PEM) is said to be a problem at ages 6 months to 2 years. Thus, this age period is considered a window period during which it is essential to prevent and/or manage acute and chronic malnutrition manifestations [4–6]. Child and maternal malnutrition together have contributed to 3.5 million annual deaths. Furthermore, children less than 5 years of age have a disease burden of 35% [7]. In 2008, 8.8 million global deaths in children less than 5 years old were due to underweight, of which 93% occurred in Africa and Asia. Approximately one in every seven children faces mortality before their fifth birthday in sub Saharan Africa (SSA) due to malnutrition [8].

Young malnourished children are affected by compromised immune systems by succumbing to infectious diseases and are prone to cognitive development delays, damaging long term psychological and intellectual development effects, as well as mental and physical development that is compromised due to stunting [7, 9–11]. A malnutrition cycle exists in populations experiencing chronic undernutrition and in this cycle, the nutritional requirements are not met in pregnant women. Thus, infants born to these mothers are of low birth weight, are unable to reach their full growth potential and may therefore be stunted, susceptible to infections, illness, and mortality early in life. The cycle is aggravated when low birth weight females grow into malnourished children and adults, and are therefore more likely to give birth to infants of low birth weight as well [9]. Malnutrition is not just a health issue but also affects the global burden of malnutrition socially, economically, developmentally and medically, affecting individuals, their families and communities with serious and long lasting consequences [1].

Studies in Sudan, Ethiopia, Bangladesh, and Haiti have indicated that the causes of malnutrition are multi-faceted, with both environmental and dietary factors contributing to malnutrition risk in young children [12]. Diet and disease have been identified as primary immediate determinants; with household food security, access to health facilities, healthy environment, and childcare practices influenced by socio-economic conditions [13]. Mother's antenatal visit and body mass index were also identified as risk factors for malnutrition [14]. In children under 3 years of age some of the main factors included poor nutrition, feeding practices, education and occupation of parent/caregiver, residence, household income, nutrition knowledge of mother [15]. These studies have suggested that nutrition education for the mother is important, as it is a resource that mothers can utilize for better care of their children. It can also provide the necessary skills required for childcare, improvement of her feeding practices, enable her to make choices and have preference of health facilities available, increase her nutritional needs awareness, and give her the chance of changing her beliefs regarding medicine and disease [16]. Some of the nutritional interventions that have had some success in addressing malnutrition include exclusive breastfeeding for the first 6 months of life, vitamin A supplementation, deworming, zinc treatment and rehydration salts for diarrhea, food fortification, and folic acid/iron for lactating and pregnant women, improvement of access to piped water and hygiene [17]. These interventions have positively influenced the development, growth and survival of children [18]. Malnutrition is not a uniform condition and therefore groups and areas that experience high risk of malnutrition must be identified and targeted interventions available to assist [17].

To determine both over and undernutrition, assessment of the nutritional status is important. This identifies those individuals who are vulnerable and at risk, and how to guide a response [19]. In determining the nutritional status of a child, it must be referenced in comparison to a healthy child [20]. Most of the anthropometric indices are used with reference tables such as that of the National Center for Health Statistics (NCHS) and the currently widely recommended and used 2006 WHO child growth standards [21]. In expressing anthropometric indices relative to a reference population, the measurements are developed using the median and standard deviations of the reference populations, which are known as Z scores [22–24]. The Z score classification system interprets weight for age (W/A), weight for height (W/H) and height for age (H/A). Z scores describe a child's mid upper arm circumference (MUAC)/weight/height in comparison to the median and the mid upper arm circumference (MUAC)/weight/height of the child relative to the reference population [25]. The anthropometric value is expressed by the two score system as "a number of standard deviations or Z scores below or above the reference mean or median value" [26]. Thus, the Z score is calculated as follows:

$$\text{Z score} = \frac{\text{observed value} - \text{median value of the reference population}}{\text{standard deviation value of reference population}} \tag{1}$$

2. Classification of malnutrition

As previously mentioned malnutrition consists of both over and undernutrition (**Table 1**).

2.1 Undernutrition

Undernutrition does not only affect the health of individuals but impacts greatly on the growth of the economy and productivity, as well as the eradication of poverty. To support their growth and development, infants and young children have increased nutritional needs and therefore are most affected by undernutrition [27, 28]. Prolonged malnourished status in children can lead to the development of

Classification	Z score values
Adequately nourished	−2 < Z-score < +1
Moderately malnourished	−3 < Z-score < −2
Severely malnourished	Z-score < −3

Table 1.
Malnutrition classification of children based on Z scores [20].

motor function and physical growth delays, lack of social skills, and low infection resistance, thus making them susceptible to common ailments and infections [28, 29]. Additionally, due to frequent infection, susceptible children become engaged in a negative cycle whereby infections lead to growth delays and their learning abilities are hindered, and infections in malnourished children may lead to childhood mortality [30].

Undernutrition is subdivided into two categories that include micronutrient malnutrition and growth failure. To differentiate between acute or chronic malnutrition, the nutritional status of an individual is assessed by using anthropometry [27]. According to Zere and McIntyre [31], anthropometry is advantageous over biochemical evaluation, as it is less invasive and cost effective; hence, in addressing child survival nutritional status anthropometry is one of the favored predictors [32]. To assess the growth status of children the most common indices used in anthropometry include low weight for height or wasting, stunting or low height for age, underweight or a low weight for age and waist/arm circumference.

2.2 Undernutrition/protein energy malnutrition (PEM)

In PEM the condition is characterized by the individual being susceptible to infection due to long-term consumption of protein and energy that is insufficient to meet the body's needs. While the body may first attempt to utilize the nutrients to meet the energy demands, if there is insufficient intake of energy then the consumed protein is used to meet the energy demands and does not address the functions of the protein in the body, hence leading to PEM. While PEM requires the measuring of growth parameters such as height and weight as it is not immediately obvious, in severe PEM children present with marasmus and kwashiorkor [33, 34]. Marasmus is characterized by a lack of protein and energy in the diet, while an inadequate intake of protein causes kwashiorkor. Marasmus or severe wasting (below −3SD) presents with a MUAC less than 115 mm in children under age five. Children with marasmus present with an "old man" appearance and are very thin [33]. In kwashiorkor, a child does not necessarily appear as undernourished but there is the presence of oedema. The children present with hair that is discolored and skin that is shiny and very tight. The weight for height is greater than or equal to −2SD. In marasmic-kwashiorkor bilateral oedema is present, with a weight for height less than −2SD [33–35].

2.3 Underweight (weight for age or W/A)

A common presentation of PEM in children is underweight. Underweight is seen as children having a weight for age with a Z score of −2SD, with severe underweight at −3SD [36, 37]. Since proteins and/or energy are insufficient in a diet, there is weight loss or failure to gain weight. This can be accompanied by a decline in linear height [38]. While the children may present with normal body proportions such as weight to height ratios, they will be undersized and underweight [39]. Through regular monitoring of growth indices such as height and weight, underweight can be identified at an early stage [26–39]. In 2013, 99 million children less than 5 years of age were underweight. Of this figure, one third of the children were from Africa and two-thirds present in Asia. An estimated 14.6% of newborns were with low birth weight in 2015, and approximately nine out of 10 of the newborns were from low and middle income countries (LMICs). Approximately 45% of deaths in LMICs in children under age five is due to underweight. In adolescent girls the underweight prevalence increased from 5.5% in 2000 to 5.7% in 2016 [40].

2.4 Stunting (height for age or H/A)

Stunting is a major public health concern that begins in intrauterine life although children are only classified as stunted at approximately age 2 years. The detrimental effects of stunting include intrauterine growth retardation, as well as inadequate nutrition required for growth and development of children [41]. High frequency of infection and decreased disease resistance such as diarrhea and pneumonia are influenced by stunting. Childhood stunting may also lead to increased mortality, poor recovery from disease and is also an obesity risk factor in adulthood [41, 42]. Stunting causes growth impairment during childhood that is associated with increased cardio-metabolic disease and obesity risk and cognitive development delay in adulthood [43]. This creates both short and long term effects that indicate the importance of stunting being identified and monitored in early life [42].

In children the initial 1000 days of life are an important window period for intervention implementation and tracking for the improvement of child growth and development [7–44]. Often stunting is correlated with poor socio-economic status, as well as environmental conditions surveys in South Africa (SA) have identified an increased stunting prevalence in black people compared to their Indian or white counterparts [31]. Some surveys looked at a wider age range of children (0–14 years) and higher stunting prevalence was found in children living informal settlements within urban and rural areas [36–45].

In stunting or low height for age the Z score is below 2 standard deviations [21]. It is prevalent usually in infants and children younger than 5 years [36], who are susceptible to infection and have an insufficient intake of nutrients over the long term. Low height for age is seen as the failure of an individual to reach full linear growth and if stunting occurs before age two then irreversible poor cognitive and motor developments may occur [41]. Severe stunting is indicated by a height for age that is lesser than the median by 85% to represent a standard deviation of −3SD [46]. In 2013 in children under 5 years of age, 161 million were identified as stunted globally. The trend of global decrease were evident from the period 2000–2013, during which figures declined from 199 million to 161 million (33–25%). However, one third of stunted children were still found in Africa [47]. During 2000–2018 the number and proportion of stunted children under age five rose by 6.5 million in Central and Western Africa and by 1.4 million in Southern and Eastern Africa. Thus, the stunting burden continues to escalate in Africa, creating serious human capital development complications [40].

2.5 Overweight and obesity

In the last five decades overweight and obesity appears to be reaching epidemic levels in both developing and developed countries [48, 49]. Eclipsing infectious disease and under-nutrition as a significant mortality and ill-health contributor, overweight and obesity have presented as the most prevalent global nutritional problem over the last two decades. Globally an estimated 1 billion adults are overweight, with 300 million of them being obese [49]. An estimated 155 million obese children contribute to this epidemic [50]. Obese children tend to become obese adults. Obesity-related health problems occur in early years of life and progress into adulthood [51]. Several chronic disease conditions in later life are associated with childhood obesity. These chronic diseases include diabetes, stroke, high blood pressure, cancers and heart disease [52]. Despite the increased prevalence of overweight and obesity in children, research evaluating treatment in these age groups is minimal. Middle-income countries such as South Africa (SA), Brazil and China have increased overweight and obesity rates across all age groups and economic levels [49].

However, over the last few years overweight has increased in every continent. It has been postulated that the number of overweight children under age five will rise from over 40 million to approximately 43 million by 2025 [53]. As of 2018, approximately half of the overweight under five children were in Asia, with a quarter in Africa. Between 2000 and 2018 in Africa, the number of overweight under five children rose by just under 44%. In children and adolescents aged 5–19 years old, the proportion of overweight in 2000 rose from one in 10 (10.3%) to just under one in five (18.4%) in 2016 [40].

2.6 Stunting versus overweight/obesity

Some developing countries such as SA are currently facing a nutrition transition with the dual burden of over and undernutrition. This nutrition transition is the replacement of traditional home cooked balanced diet meals by energy-dense foods, as well as sedentary lifestyles due to technology and urbanization. A review study highlighted the dual burden in SA in children aged 0–20 years. The prevalence of wasting and stunting was higher in younger male children and predominant in rural areas, whereas overweight/obesity prevalence was highest in females and children in urban settings. It is important for tracking of over and undernutrition in children at a district level that can also be used to prioritize, monitor and evaluate government policies regarding malnutrition [54]. More recent years have seen the double burden of malnutrition being accompanied by a triple burden of malnutrition, affecting families, communities and countries. In countries such as India and Egypt, the problem is increasing and therefore highlights the urgent need to consider child malnutrition in the greater familial and household contexts [40–55]. A study in Ghana addressed the concurrent occurrence of obesity and stunting in children aged under 5 years, providing data for the first time on such an occurrence. The study reported a stunting prevalence of 27.5%, overweight prevalence of 2.4% and an overall concurrent stunting and overweight prevalence of 1.2% [56]. A study in South Africa, with children aged 6–12 years old, reported that 9.1% were stunted, while 14.9% were overweight/obese [57]. This highlights the need for urgent targeted interventions in children to address this double burden to prevent these malnutrition issues as they transition into adulthood.

2.7 Wasting (weight for length/height or W/H)

In wasting or low weight for height the Z score is below 2 standard deviations [21]. Wasting is reflective of a body mass that is low in comparison to the age and may be due to disease or starvation. Weight loss and retardation of growth occur due to inadequate intake of food and long term it leads to wasting and becomes more severe with emaciation [58]. A child falls behind another child who is growing actively when his/her own growth is affected acutely [38], and the body height and weight become less than ideal for the age of the child [59]. Severe wasting occurs when the weight for height is less than the median by 70% to represent a standard deviation of −3SD [46]. According to the national Department of Health (DoH) height measurements in all children should be conducted at least every 3 months [60]. In measuring overall growth to compare growth standards, both height and weight measurements are essential. Globally, in 2013, in children less than 5 years of age, 51 million were wasted and 17 million severely wasted. Global wasting prevalence in 2013 approximated 8%, of which 3% accounted for severe wasting. A postulated third of wasted children were present in Africa and an estimate of the children severely wasted in Africa followed the same trend [61]. As of 2018–2019 52 million children are wasted, with an estimated 16.6 suffering from severe wasting in

2018 [62]. Children left untreated with severe acute malnutrition (SAM) are at least 12 times more likely to die than healthy children [63]. South Asia is the global wasting epicenter as 15.2% of children under five are wasted. Together with other hotspots such as Oceania, Southeast Asia and SSA, improvements regarding wasting are minimal [64] (**Table 2**).

Country	Year of last survey	Wasting	Overweight	Stunting	Underweight
Angola	2015–2016	4.9	3.4	37.6	19.0
Benin	2017–2018	5.0	1.9	32.2	16.8
Botswana	2007–2008	7.2	11.2	31.4	11.2
Burkina Faso	2017	8.6	1.7	21.1	16.2
Burundi	2016–2017	5.1	1.4	55.9	29.3
Cabo Verde	1994	6.9	—	21.4	11.8
Cameroon	2014	5.2	6.7	31.7	14.8
Central African Republic	2012	7.6	1.9	39.6	24.6
Chad	2014–2015	13.3	2.8	39.8	29.4
Comoros	2012	11.3	10.6	31.1	16.9
The Congo	2014–2015	8.2	5.9	21.2	12.3
Cote d'Ivoire	2016	6.1	1.5	21.6	12.8
Democratic Republic of Congo	2013–2014	8.1	4.4	42.7	23.4
Djibouti	2012	21.6	8.1	33.5	29.9
Equatorial Guinea	2011	3.1	9.7	26.2	5.6
Eritrea	2010	15.3	2.0	52.0	39.4
Eswatini (former Swaziland)	2014	2.0	9.0	25.5	5.8
Ethiopia	2016	10.0	2.9	38.4	23.6
Gabon	2012	3.4	7.7	17.0	6.4
The Gambia	2013	11.0	3.2	24.6	16.5
Ghana	2014	4.7	2.6	18.8	11.2
Guinea	2016	8.1	4.0	32.4	18.3
Guinea—Bissau	2014	6.0	2.3	27.6	17.0
Kenya	2014	4.2	4.1	26.2	11.2
Lesotho	2014	2.8	7.5	33.4	10.5
Liberia	2013	5.6	3.2	32.1	15.3
Madagascar	2012–2013	7.9	1.1	48.9	32.9
Malawi	2015–2016	2.8	4.6	37.4	11.8
Mali	2015	13.5	1.9	30.4	25.0
Mauritania	2015	14.8	1.3	27.9	24.9
Mauritius	1995	15.7	6.5	13.6	13.0
Mozambique	2011	6.1	7.8	42.9	15.6
Namibia	2013	7.1	4.0	22.7	13.2

Country	Year of last survey	Wasting	Overweight	Stunting	Underweight
Niger	2016	10.1	1.1	40.6	31.4
Nigeria	2016–2017	10.8	1.5	43.6	31.5
Rwanda	2014–2015	2.3	7.9	38.2	9.6
Sao Tome and Principe	2014	4.0	2.4	17.2	8.8
Senegal	2017	9.0	0.9	16.5	14.4
Seychelles	2012	4.3	10.2	7.9	3.6
Sierra Leone	2013	9.5	8.8	37.8	18.2
Somalia	2009	15.0	3.0	25.3	23.0
South Africa	2016	2.5	13.3	27.4	5.9
South Sudan	2010	24.3	5.8	31.3	29.1
Togo	2013–2014	6.6	2.0	27.6	16.1
Uganda	2016	3.5	3.7	28.9	10.4
United Republic of Tanzania	2015–16	4.5	3.7	34.5	13.7
Zambia	2013–14	6.2	6.2	40.0	14.9
Zimbabwe	2015	3.3	5.6	27.1	8.5

Table 2.
Joint malnutrition country estimates of anthropometric indicators in children aged 0–59 months [65].

3. Malnutrition in South Africa

As a developing or middle-income country, SA is still undergoing major transitions socially, economically and in the population's health. The country is currently facing a quadruple disease burden, with non-communicable diseases linked to diet and lifestyle; the burden of Human Immunodeficiency Virus/Acquired immunodeficiency syndrome (HIV/AIDS); infectious diseases and poverty linked to under nutrition; and deaths due to injuries [66]. As a developing country SA is in a nutrition transition where both over and undernutrition coexist [67]. The first 2 years of life are a vulnerable time frame as it is during this period that malnutrition begins. According to Faber and Wenhold [68], chronic malnutrition or stunting is more prevalent in children in SA compared to wasting. Since the post-apartheid era in 1994, SA has faced great challenges in addressing the nutritional status of infants, young children and adults [69]. However, large-scale nationwide surveys were conducted to trace the progress, failures and successes in addressing malnutrition. In 1994 the South African Vitamin A Consultative Group (SAVACG) conducted a national survey on the nutritional status of children aged 6–71 months [70]. Anthropometric results revealed that approximately 10% or 660,000 children were underweight, with one in every four children (1.5 million) affected by stunting. Severe wasting was only recorded in 0.4% of children. KwaZulu-Natal (KZN), Eastern Cape and Northern Province revealed the greatest prevalence of malnutrition [70]. In 1999 the National Food Consumption Survey (NFCS) was conducted in children aged 1–9 years [71], collecting a larger set of data in comparison to the SAVACG survey. The NFCS reported 10% underweight in children, with 20% affected by stunting and 17.1% as overweight and/or obese. The NFCS secondary analysis, focusing on children aged 1–5 years, reported underweight at 6.8%, stunting at 20.1%, overweight at 20.6% and obesity at 9.5% [69]. In 2005, the

National Food Consumption Survey-Fortification Baseline (NFCS-FB) reported that of children aged 1–9 years old, 20% were affected by stunting, 9.3% were underweight, wasting was found in 4.5%, and 14% were overweight or obese [72]. The South African National Health and Nutrition Examination Survey (SANHANES) conducted in 2012 reported that in children aged 0–14 years stunting prevalence was 15.4%, with 3.8% having severe stunting. Wasting was reported at 2.9%, with severe wasting at 0.8%. Underweight was reported at 5.8%, with severe underweight at 1.1%. Regarding over nutrition, SANHANES identified 18.1% of children as overweight and 4.6% as obese [36]. The prevalence of overweight and obesity was significantly greater in females (25% and 40.1%) compared to males (19.6% and 11.6%) respectively. Underweight was significantly higher in males (13.1%) in comparison to females (4.0%) [36]. Thus, it is evident that SA is facing the malnutrition epidemic at a young age and context-specific and targeted interventions are required to prevent child malnutrition before it progresses into adulthood.

4. Conclusion

During 2012–2013, WHO member states recognized the seriousness of malnutrition and its effect on global health [3]. Thus, at the United Nation's General Assembly in 2016, the United Nations Decade of Action on Nutrition 2016–2025 was announced. This set a time frame for all forms of malnutrition to be addressed and for diet-related and nutrition targets to be met by 2025. This also set the time frame for the Sustainable Development Goals (SGDs) to be achieved before 2030, particularly SDG 2 that aims to improve nutrition, achieve food security and end hunger, as well as SDG 3 that aims to ensure healthy living and promote well-being for all [1]. To tackle the malnutrition epidemic food fortification is important to ensure that children with good weight do not risk becoming overweight or obese [73]. All malnutrition indicators must be included in interventions, and more importantly treated together rather than stand-alone issues [74]. As part of the health system strengthening and with the goal of combatting malnutrition, existing policies on child malnutrition must be evaluated. The coexistence of stunting and overweight/obesity remains a challenge in LMICs that requires multi-sectoral action. During infancy and early childhood optimal nutrition is vital to ensure that, development and rapid growth demands are met. In the efforts to tackle the nutrition disparities, the first 1000 days of life are an important window period, presenting the opportunity to prevent both stunting and overweight/obesity [75]. Interventions must be inclusive of both linear growth and appropriate weight, beginning in early life and preferably during this important window period. To further tackle the double and triple burdens of malnutrition, early screening and identification of at risk children, including those already with malnutrition, is essential at healthcare facilities [76]. Thus, a more holistic, context-specific approach is required, whereby interventions not only take into consideration the risk factors, but also consider the inclusion of nutritionists and educating mothers on self and childcare regarding nutrition [77]. Furthermore, child malnutrition research and interventions must be up-scaled from community level to provincial and national levels so that it informs policy on the intervention strategies that can address the burden of child malnutrition. This is vital as children left untreated transition into malnourished adulthood, increasing the healthcare costs and needs, weakening the healthcare systems, and perpetuating the vicious malnutrition cycle.

Author details

Natisha Dukhi
Human Sciences Research Council, Cape Town, South Africa

*Address all correspondence to: doctordukhi@gmail.com

References

[1] World Health Organization (WHO). Malnutrition [Internet] 2019. Available from: https://www.who.int/news-room/fact-sheets/detail/malnutrition

[2] World Health Organization (WHO). Nutrition [Internet] 2020. Available from: https://www.who.int/nutrition/topics/2_background/en/index1.html

[3] Global Nutrition Report 2018 [Internet]. 2018. Available from: https://globalnutritionreport.org/reports/global-nutrition-report-2018/

[4] Shrimpton R, Victora CG, De Onis M, Lima RC, Blossner M, Clugston G. Worldwide timing of growth faltering: Implications for nutritional interventions. Paediatrics. 2001;**107**(5):75-81. DOI: 10.1542/peds.107.5.e75

[5] Bern C, Nathanail L. Is mid-upper-arm circumference a useful tool for screening in emergency settings? Lancet. 1995;**345**:631-633. DOI: 10.1016/s0140-6736(95)90527-8

[6] Benson T. Improving Nutrition as a Development Priority: Addressing Undernutrition in National Policy Processes in Sub-Saharan Africa [Internet]. Washington DC: International Food Policy Research Institute; 2008. Available from: http://www.ifpri.org/sites/default/files/publications/rr156.pdf

[7] Black RE, Allen LH, Bhutta ZA, Caulfield LE, de Onis M, Ezzati M. Maternal and child undernutrition: Global and regional exposures and health consequences. Lancet. 2008;**371**:243-260. DOI: 10.1016/S0140-6736(07)61690-0

[8] Walton E, Allen S. Malnutrition in developing countries. Paediatrics and Child Health. 2011;**21**(9):418-424. DOI: 10.1016/j.paed.2011.04.004

[9] Nutrition and South Africa's Children [Internet]. nd. Available from: http://www.soulcity.org.za/projects/soul-buddyz/soul-buddyz-series-3/literature-review/nutrition-literature-review

[10] Blössner M, DeOnis M. Malnutrition: Quantifying the health impact at national and local levels. In: Environmental Burden of Disease Series [Internet]. 2005. p. 12. Available from: https://apps.who.int/iris/handle/10665/43120

[11] Grantham-McGregor S. A review of studies of the effect of severe malnutrition on mental development. Journal of Nutrition. 1995;**125**(8):2233S-2238S

[12] De Onis M, Monteiro C, Akre J, et al. The worldwide magnitude of protein energy malnutrition; an overview from the WHO global database on child growth. Bulletin of the World Health Organization. 1993;**71**:703-712

[13] Müller O, Krawinkel M. Malnutrition and health in developing countries. CMAJ. 2005;**173**:279-286. DOI: 10.1503/cmaj.050342

[14] Siddiqi NA, Haque N, Goni MA. Malnutrition of under-five children: Evidence from Bangladesh. Asian Journal of Medical Sciences. 2001;**2**:113-118. DOI: 10.3126/ajms.v2i2.3662

[15] Seligman HK, Laraia BA, Kushel MB. Food insecurity is associated with chronic disease among low-income NHANES participants. The Journal of Nutrition. 2010;**140**:304-310. DOI: 10.3945/jn.109.112573

[16] Tesfaye M. Bayesian approach to identify predictors of children Nutritional status in Ethiopia [thesis] [Internet]. 2009. Available from: http://localhost:80/xmlui/handle/123456789/4465

[17] Ayoya AM, Heidkamp R, Ngnie, Teta I, Pierre JM, Stoltzfus RJ. Child malnutrition in Haiti: Progress despite disasters. Global Health: Science and Practice. 2013;**1**(3):389-396. DOI: 10.9745/GHSP-D-13-00069

[18] Bhutta ZA, Das JK, Rizvi A, Gaffey MF, Walker N, Horton S, et al. Evidence-based interventions for improvement of maternal and child nutrition: What can be done and at what cost? Lancet. 2013;**382**(9890):452-477. DOI: 10.1016/S0140-6736(13)60996-4

[19] Pan American Health Organization. Understanding Malnutrition [Internet]. 2013. Available from: https://cursos.campusvirtualsp.org/pluginfile.php/73101/mod_resource/content/6/Unit%202%20–%20Understanding%20malnutrition.pdf

[20] Webb P and Bhatia RA. A Manual: Measuring and Interpreting Malnutrition and Mortality [Internet]. 2005. Available from: http://www.unhcr.org/45f6abc92.html

[21] World Health Organization (WHO). WHO Child Growth Standards: Length/Height-for-Age, Weight-for-Age, Weight-for-Length, Weight-for-Height and Body Mass Index-for-Age: Methods and Development [Internet]. Geneva: World Health Organization; 2006. Available from: https://www.who.int/childgrowth/standards/technical_report/en/

[22] Jellife DB. The assessment of the nutritional status of the community. In: WHO Monographs [Internet]. 1966. p. 53. Available from: https://apps.who.int/iris/handle/10665/41780

[23] Sachdev HPS. Assessment of nutritional status. Bulletin of the World Health Organization. 1977;**55**(1):489-498

[24] Waterlow JC, Buzina RKW, Lane JM, Nichaman MZ, Tanner JM. The presentation and use of height and weight data for comparing the nutritional status of children under the age of 10 years. Bulletin of the World Health Organization. 1977;**55**(4):489-498

[25] Pederson D, Gore C. Anthropometry Measurement Error. Sydney, Australia: University of New South Wales Press; 1996

[26] World Health Organization (WHO). WHO global database on child growth and malnutrition. In: World Health Organization/Programme of Nutrition [Internet]. 2004. Available from: http://www.who.int/nutgrowthdb/en/

[27] Torún B. Protein-Energy Malnutrition in, Modern Nutrition in Health and Disease. United States of America: Lippincott Williams & Wilkins; 2006

[28] Fentahun W, Wubshet M, Tariku A. Undernutrition and associated factorsamong children aged 6-59 months in east Belesa District, Northwest Ethiopia: A community based cross-sectional study. BMC Public Health. 2016;**16**(506):1-10. DOI: 10.1186/s12889-016-3180-0

[29] Kandala NB, Madungu TP, Emina JBO, Nzita KPD, Cappuccio FP. Malnutrition among children under the age of five in the Democratic Republic of Congo (DRC): Does geographic location matter? BMC Public Health. 2011;**11**(261):1-15. DOI: 10.1186/1471-2458-11-261

[30] Mengistu K, Alemu K, Destaw B. Prevalence of malnutrition and associated factors among children aged 6-59 months at Hidabu Abote District, North Shewa Oromia Regional State. Journal of Nutritional Disorders and Therapy. 2013;**1**(1):1-15. DOI: 10.4172/2161-0509.1000T1-001

[31] Zere E, McIntyre D. Inequities in under-five child malnutrition in South

Africa. International Journal for Equity in Health. 2003;**2**(7). DOI: 10.1186/1475-9276-2-7

[32] National Department of Health: Directorate Nutrition. The Integrated Nutrition Programme—Nutritional Status [Internet]. 2005. Available from: http://www.doh.gov.za/programmes/inp/status.html

[33] Taking Action, Nutrition for Survival, Growth & Development ACF International White Paper [Internet]. 2010. Available from: http://www.actionagainsthunger.org.uk/resource-centre/online-library/detail/media/acf-international-white-paper/

[34] Sisodia U, Desai N, Akerkar S. Protein energy malnutrition severe acute malnutrition, LRTI with KOCH'S. Acta Scientific Nutritional Health. 2018; **2**(5):19-20

[35] Save the Children. Emergency Health and Nutrition [Internet]. 2014. Available from: https://www.savethechildren.org/us/what-we-do/global-programs/health/health-and-nutrition-emergencies

[36] Shisana O, Labadarios D, Rehle T, Simbayi L, Zuma K, Dhansay A, et al. South African National Health and Nutrition Examination Survey (SANHANES-1): Edition. Cape Town: HSRC Press; 2014

[37] Wittenberg DF. Nutritional Disorders. Oxford: South Africa; 2004

[38] Golden MHN, Golden BE. Severe Malnutrition in Human Nutrition and Dietetics. United Kingdom: Churchill Livingstone; 2000

[39] United Nations Children's Fund (UNICEF). CHILDINFO: Monitoring the Situation of Children and Women. United Nations Children's Fund [Internet]. 2009. Available from: http://www.childinfo.org/files/MICS3_Chapter_0- Title_Page_and_Contents.pdf

[40] United Nations Children's Fund (UNICEF). The State of the World's Children 2019. Children, Food and Nutrition: Growing Well in a Changing World [Internet]. 2019. Available from: https://www.unicef.org/reports/state-of-worlds-children-2019

[41] Mzumara B, Bwembya P, Halwiindi H, Mugode R, Banda J. Factors associated with stunting among children below five years of age in Zambia: Evidence from the 2014 Zambia demographic and health survey. BMC Nutrition. 2018;**4**(51):1-8. DOI: 10.1186/s40795-018-0260-9

[42] Pelletier DL, Frongillo EA Jr, Schroeder DG, Habicht JP. The effects of malnutrition on child mortality in developing counties. Bulletin of the World Health Organization. 1995;**73**: 443-448

[43] Victora CG, Adair L, Fall C, Hallal PC, Martorell R, Richter L, et al. Maternal and child undernutrition: Consequences for adult health and human capital. Lancet. 2008;**371**: 340-357. DOI: 10.1016/S0140-6736(07)61692-4

[44] Prentice AM, Ward KA, Goldberg GR, Jarjou LM, Moore SE, Fulford AJ, et al. Critical windows for nutritional interventions against stunting. The American Journal of Clinical Nutrition. 2013;**97**(5):911-918. DOI: 10.3945/ajcn.112.052332

[45] Ardington C, Case A. Health: Analysis of the National Income Dynamics Study (NIDS) Wave 1 Dataset. Cape Town: Southern Africa Labour and Development Research Unit, School of Economics, University of Cape Town [Internet]; 2009. Available from: https://pdfs.semanticscholar.org/f693/a6d90fb4a895c84f609589fa6148f2c20db1.pdf

[46] Picot J, Hartwell D, Harris P, Mendes D, Clegg AJ, Takeda A. The effectiveness of interventions to treat severe acute malnutrition in young children: A systematic review. Health Technology Assessment. 2012;**16**(19). DOI: 10.3310/hta16190

[47] United Nations Children's Fund (UNICEF). State of the World's Children. Maternal and Newborn Health [Internet]. 2009. Available from: http://www.unicef.org/sowc09/

[48] Müller MJ, Asbeck I, Mast M, Largnäse K, Grund A. Prevention of obesity—more than an intention. Concept and first results of the Kiel Obesity Prevention Study (KOPS). International Journal of Obesity. 2001;**25**(1):S66-S74. DOI: 10.1038/sj.ijo.0801703

[49] Kruger HS, Puoane T, Senekal M, van der Merwe MT. Obesity in South Africa: Challenges for government and health professionals. Public Health Nutrition. 2005;**8**(5):491-500. DOI: 10.1079/PHN2005785

[50] Hossain P, Kawar B, El Nahas M. Obesity and diabetes in the developing world—A growing challenge. The New England Journal of Medicine. 2007;**356**: 3. DOI: 10.1056/NEJMp068177

[51] Lau DCW, Douketis JD, Morrison KM, Hramiak IM, Sharma AM, Ur E. 2006 Canadian clinical practice guidelines on the management and prevention of obesity in adults and children (summary). Canadian Medical Association Journal. 2007;**176**(8):S1-S13. DOI: 10.1503/cmaj.061409

[52] Brennan L, Walkley J, Fraser SF, Greenway K, Wilks R. Motivational interviewing and cognitive behaviour therapy in the treatment of adolescent overweight and obesity: Study design and methodology. Contemporary Clinical Trials. 2008;**29**:359-375. DOI: 10.1016/j.cct.2007.09.001

[53] UNICEF, WHO, International Bank for Reconstruction and Development and World Bank. Levels and Trends in Child Malnutrition: Key Findings of the 2019 Edition of the Joint Child Malnutrition Estimates [Internet]. Geneva: WHO; 2019. Available from: https://www.who.int/nutgrowthdb/estimates2018/en/

[54] Stevens G, Finucane M, Paciorek C, Flaxman S, White R, Donner A, et al. Nutrition Impact Model Study Group. Trends in mild, moderate, and severe stunting and underweight, and progress towards MDG 1 in 141 developing countries: A systematic analysis of population representative data. Lancet. 2012;**380**:824-834. DOI: 10.1016/S0140-6736(12)60647-3

[55] Dang A, Meenakshi JV. The nutrition transition and the intra-household double burden of malnutrition in India. In: ADBI Working Paper 725 [Internet]. Tokyo: Asian Development Bank Institute; 2017. Available from: https://www.adb.org/publications/nutrition-transition-household-malnutrition-india

[56] Atsu BK, Guure C, Laar AK. Determinants of overweight with concurrent stunting among Ghanaian children. BMC Pediatrics. 2017;**17**(177): 1-12. DOI: 10.1186/s12887-017-0928-3

[57] Graham L, Hochfeld T, Stuart L. Double trouble: Addressing stunting and obesity via school nutrition. South African journal of child health. 2018; **12**(3):90-94. DOI: 10.7196/SAJCH.2018.v12i3.1455

[58] Briend, Khara T, Dolan C. Wasting and stunting—Similarities and differences: Policy and programmatic implications. Food and Nutrition Bulletin. 2015;**36**(1):S15-S23

[59] Shetty P. Food and Nutrition: The Global Challenge. United Kingdom: Blackwell Publishing; 2002

[60] National Department of Health. National Guidelines on Nutrition for People Living with HIV, AIDS, TB and Other Chronic Debilitating Conditions. South Africa: Department of Health; 2007

[61] United Nations Children's Fund, World Health Organization, The World Bank. UNICEFWHO-World Bank Joint Child Malnutrition Estimates [Internet]. New York; Geneva; Washington, DC: UNICEF; WHO; The World Bank; 2012. Available from: http://www.who.int/nutgrowthdb/jme_unicef_who_wb.pdf

[62] No Wasted Lives Coalition (undated). State of acute malnutrition. In: UNICEF, WHO and World Bank Group. Joint Child Malnutrition Estimates [Internet]. Geneva: WHO; 2019. Available from: https://www.acutemalnutrition.org/en/countries

[63] Olofin I et al. Associations of suboptimal growth with all-cause and cause specific mortality in children under five years: A pooled analysis of ten prospective studies'. PLoS One. 2013;**8**(5):e64636. DOI: 10.1371/journal.pone.0064636

[64] Harding KL, Aguayo VM, Webb P. Factors associated with wasting among children under five years old in South Asia: Implications for action. PLoS One. 2018;**13**(7):e0198749

[65] United Nations Children's Fund (UNICEF). Malnutrition [Internet]. 2019. Available from: https://data.unicef.org/topic/nutrition/malnutrition/

[66] Steyn NP, Bradshaw D, Norman R, Joubert J, Schneider M, Steyn K. Dietary Changes and The Health Transition in South Africa: Implications for Health Policy [Internet]. Cape Town: South African Medical Research Council; 2006. Available from: http://www.fao.org/docrep/009/a0442e/a0442e0v.html

[67] Combating malnutrition in South Africa. Input Paper for Health Roadmap [Internet] 2008. Available from: http://www.dbsa.org/EN/AboutUs/Publications/Documents/South%20Africa%20Nutrition_%20input%20paper_roadmap.pdf

[68] Faber M, Wenhold F. Nutrition in contemporary South Africa. Water South Africa. 2007;**33**(3):393-399. DOI: 10.4314/wsa.v33i3.49122

[69] Iversen PO, du Plessis L, Marais D, Morseth M, Høisæther EA. Nutritional health of young children in South Africa over the first 16 years of democracy. SAJCH. 2011;**5**(3):72-77. DOI: http://hdl.handle.net/10019.1/19087

[70] Labadarios D, Van Middelkoop A, The South African Vitamin A Consultative Group (SAVACG). Children Aged 6 to 71 Months in South Africa, 1994: Their Anthropometric, Vitamin a, Iron and Immunisation Coverage Status. Isando: SAVACG. 1995

[71] Labadarios D, Steyn NP, Maunder E, et al. The National Food Consumption Survey (NFCS): South Africa, 1999. Public Health Nutrition. 2005;**8**:533-543

[72] Labadarios D. National Food Consumption Survey-Fortification Baseline (NFCS-FB): South Africa 2005 [Internet]. Pretoria: Directorate: Nutrition, Department of Health; 2007. Available from: http://www.sajcn.co.za/index.php/SAJCN/article/view/286

[73] Rachmi CN, Agho KE, Li M, Baur LA. Stunting, underweight and overweight in children aged 2.0–4.9 years in Indonesia: Prevalence trends and associated risk factors. PLoS One. 2016;**11**(5):e0154756. DOI: 10.1371/journal.pone.0154756

[74] Shrimpton R, Rokx C. The Double Burden of Malnutrition in Indonesia. Jakarta, Indonesia: World Bank Jakarta. Contract No.: Report 76192-ID [Internet]; 2013. Available from: http://documents.worldbank.org/curated/en/

955671468049836790/The-double-burden-of-malnutrition-in-Indonesia

[75] Perez-Escamilla R, Bermudez O, Buccini GS, Kumanyika S, Lutter CK, Monsivais P, et al. Nutrition disparities and the global burden of malnutrition. BMJ. 2018;**361**:1-8. DOI: 10.1136/bmj.k2252

[76] Steenkamp L, Lategan R, Raubenheimer J. Moderate malnutrition in children aged five years and younger in South Africa: Are wasting or stunting being treated? South African Journal of Clinical Nutrition. 2016;**29**(1):27-31 Available from: http://www.sajcn.co.za/index.php/SAJCN/article/view/1030

[77] Modjadji P, Madiba S. The double burden of malnutrition in a rural health and demographic surveillance system site in South Africa: A study of primary schoolchildren and their mothers. BMC Public Health. 2019;**19**(1087):1-11 . Available from. DOI: 10.1186/s12889-019-7412-y

Chapter 7

Detection of Nutrient-Related SNP to Reveal Individual Malnutrition Risk

Junsheng Huo and Chunhong Zhang

Abstract

Malnutrition is a result of complicated reasons from diet and food behavior and also related to genetic background which has been revealed by studies in recent decades. Traditionally, nutrition status are measured and expressed with indexes of anthropometric, diet survey, clinical symptom, biochemistry, behavior, etc. These measurement has been used in national nutrition monitoring, clinic nutrition therapy, mother and children nutrition care, nutrition intervention projects, and scientific studies. However, genetic and epigenetic information on nutrition explain malnutrition in a genetic view that would supply additional new theory and methodology for the growing requirement in terms of personalized and precise nutrition. In this chapter, an introduction on the detection of nutrient-related SNP to reveal individual malnutrition risk is discussed.

Keywords: SNP, nutrients, malnutrition

1. Introduction

Malnutrition is a state of disordered nutrition, in which a combination of varying degrees of over- or undernutrition and inflammatory activity has led to a change in body composition, diminished function, and outcome [1]. Malnutrition, including undernutrition, micronutrient deficiencies, and overweight and obesity, not only affects the people's health and well-being by impacting negatively on human physical and cognitive development, compromising the immune system, increasing susceptibility to communicable and noncommunicable diseases, restricting the attainment of human potential, and reducing productivity but also poses a high burden in the form of negative social and economic consequences to individuals, families, communities, and states [2].

Currently, more than 810 million people worldwide are hungry, mainly in poor, natural disaster-destroyed and war-torn countries. About 2 billion people are suffering from micronutrient deficiencies, which is called hidden hunger, and about 2 billion adults are affected by overweight and obesity, with one in 12 adults suffering from diabetes and one in two with cardiovascular diseases [3]. Developmental Origins of Health and Disease (DoHaD theory) considers that adult disease stems from malnutrition in the fetus and early childhood. More evidence accumulated that malnutrition would result in adverse consequences to the later life cycle and should be addressed in the whole life cycle [4].

Malnutrition is a result of complicated reasons from diet and food behavior and also related to genetic background which has been revealed by studies in recent decades. Traditionally, nutrition status are measured and expressed with indexes of anthropometric, diet survey, clinical symptom, biochemistry, behavior, etc. [5]. These measurement has been used in national nutrition monitoring, clinic nutrition therapy, mother and children nutrition care, nutrition intervention projects, and scientific studies. However, genetic and epigenetic information on nutrition explain malnutrition in a genetic view that would supply additional new theory and methodology for the growing requirement in terms of personalized and precise nutrition. In this chapter, an introduction on detection of nutrient-related SNP to reveal individual malnutrition risk is discussed.

2. Malnutrition related to inheritance

Following the restrictive enzyme cut technology on fragment length polymorphisms and short series repeat sequences, single nucleotide polymorphisms (SNP) became the third-generation polymorphism marker with the characteristics of high genetic marker density, high stability, and high feasibility of automation detection, which showed a strong application prospect in human genomics research, such as genetic diagnosis, genetic risk assessment, chain imbalance map, and genetic association analysis. Severe malnutrition such as iron deficiency anemia, xerophthalmia and nyctalopia, pellagra, scurvy, rickets, beriberi, and other nutrient deficiency diseases was caused by the combined impact of environment and genetic factors. And the Human Genome Project study showed that 99.9% of DNA sequences were consistent among different individuals, with only small genetic differences in the sequence. 0.1% of DNA sequence differences may vary the level of risk of malnutrition and diseases such as non-chronic diseases. Single nucleotide polymorphism could be measureable markers to reveal the genetic differences.

2.1 Iron deficiency-related genes

The discovery of polymorphisms on DNA sequences associated with common diseases was an important way to understand the risk of nutritional deficiency from genetic perspective. Iron deficiency was one of the most important nutritional problems in the world, especially in developing countries. Iron deficiency not only leads to anemia but also causes the body's immune function, work performance, and damage of adolescent's psychological behavior and mental development. With the deepening of research on nutritional genomics, genetic polymorphisms associated with iron nutrition status have been found. A study reported by Mclaren et al. [6] showed that rs2111833 and rs1121312 in TMPRSS6 gene with iron biochemical indicators showed that rs2111833 is associated with serum iron and log-to-ferritin saturation in the Caucasian population and shows total iron binding force, unsaturated iron binding force, and serum iron in the Asian population. Rs1421312 sites were associated with serum iron and log-to-ferritin saturation in the Caucasian population and serum iron and log-ferritin saturation in the Afro-American population. The study found that rs2111833 and rs1421312 had an impact on iron nutrition in different races.

3. Folic acid deficiency genes

Folic acid was a cofactor that interacted with a variety of enzymes in many intercellular reactions, with methionine enzymes acting as coenzymes when isocysteine was converted to cystic thiopental. The extent to which the body absorbed folic acid and vitamin B_6 and B_{12} is influenced by environmental and genetic factors. In 1964, Smithells et al. [7] showed that women with reproductive neural tube malformations (neural tube defect, NTD) had micronutrient deficiencies, especially folic acid. NTDs were congenital malformations of the brain and spinal cord that occurred within pregnancy from 21 to 28 days, including spina bifida, anencephaly, and brain bulging, which could lead to infant death and child disability. NTDs had the epidemiological characteristics of environmental and genetic factors. In 1995, a variant of MTHFR enzyme was identified which causes a substitution of C to T at nucleotide 677 [8]. The MTHFR C677T homozygous variant (TT genotype) is thermolabile, and its activity is reduced by 70% compared to the wild type (CC genotype). This reduced enzyme activity causes an accumulation of plasma homocysteine and higher rates of thymidylate synthesis. It is well established that B vitamin status is affected by genotype, particularly the C677T polymorphism in MTHFR, with the T allele being associated with higher circulating concentrations of homocysteine and lower circulating concentrations of plasma and erythrocyte folate. In 2018, Zhang et al. [9, 10] explored the association between maternal methylenetetrahydrofolate reductase (*MTHFR*) C677T, methionine synthase reductase (*MTRR*) A66G, and methionine synthase (*MTR*) A2756G which effects on absorption and utilization of folate, B_6 and B_{12}, and neural tube defects in offspring through meta-analysis, which showed that these SNPs were significantly associated with NTDs in offspring. A cross-sectional study of dietary and genetic predictors of blood folate levels in a large racial healthy young adults group by Daniel et al. in 2017 [11] showed that the interactive effect of the genotype with naturally occurring food folate intake on RBC folate levels occurred in the anticipated stronger individuals that is homozygous for the T allele. This pattern suggests that polyglutamated folic acid (naturally occurring food folate) is less well absorbed among C allele carriers. This interpretation is consistent with the results from previous research, which found that those with hypofunctional *FOLH1* 484 variants had lower RBC folate levels despite equivalent dietary folate intake. Understanding why circulating folate levels vary from person to person is critical to ensuring adequate bioavailability, especially among women of childbearing age.

3.1 Genes of other nutrients deficiency

In recent years, the levels of folic acid; vitamin B_2, B_3, B_6, and B_{12}; and homocysteine (HCY) in pregnant women, as well as enzymes in folic acid and HCY pathways such as methylenetetrahydrofolate reductase (MTHFR), methionine synthase reductase (MTRR), and gene polymorphism sites associated with methionine synostic ingendraase (MTR) have been explored as potential causes of NTDs. Wilcken et al. [12] showed that the frequency of the homozygous C677T genotype (TT) was highest among individuals of Hispanic ethnicity, followed by whites, with the lowest frequency found in blacks. There were geographical and racial differences in gene polymorphisms, so future studies should conduct large samples and cross-regional surveys and established a database of gene polymorphisms in different regions and populations to provide a scientific basis for precise nutrition guidance and intervention.

3.2 Measurement of malnutrition-related SNPs

Nutrigenomics studies have sufficiently accumulated data in the last two decades to reveal phenotypes of SNPs between health and micronutrient deficiency population [13]. Zhang et al. [9, 10] explored that the genes of MTHFR C677T,

MTRR A66G, and MTR A2756G were genetic factors for low absorption and bioavailability of folate, B_6, B_{12}, etc. Those nutrients are closely related with the prevalence of neural tube defects (NTDs) in newborn infants. Daniel et al. [11] reported that mutant genotype of a C allele SNP of individuals predicted lower RBC folate concentration than that of T allele SNP of individuals with the same diet folate intake level. Studies have reported numbers of micronutrient deficiency-related SNPs (MD-SNPs) of vitamins A, D, E, B_6, and B_{12}, folate, calcium, iron, zinc, selenium, etc. [14–22]. It is assumed that MD-SNPs based on high -quality observations in large population could be used as biomarkers for assessing genetic potential risk of micronutrient deficiency. The sequencing of the human genome has catalyzed efforts to search for disease genes by the strategy of associating sequence variants with measurable phenotypes. In particular, the Human Genome Project and follow-on efforts to characterize genetic variation have resulted in the discovery of millions of SNPs, which have emerged as genetic markers of choice because of their high-density and relatively even distribution in the human genomes. When one nutrient deficiency risk-related gene has been mapped to a chromosomal region, a high-density SNP mapping or candidate gene association studies are logical steps to follow.

3.3 Gene sequencing

The first-generation sequencing technology, also known as Sanger sequencing method, is based on the sequencing of DNA polymerase synthesis reaction. The basic principle is that the test DNA template, desired DNA synthase, deoxynucleoside triphosphates (dNTPs), reaction buffer, primers, and other components of DNA synthesis reaction and a small amount of four kinds of radioisotope dideoxynucleoside triphosphates (ddATP, ddTTP, ddCTP, and ddGTP) were added to the reaction system. Because the ddNTP dideoxyribose connected on the 3-carbon atom is not a hydroxyl group (-OH) but the hydrogen (H) after deoxidation, the ddNTP is added to the DNA strand being synthesized, the system subsequent to dNTP no longer be bound to this DNA strand, and the synthesis of this DNA strand was randomly terminated at the base of the ddNTP. Thus, after several cycles, a group is formed from short to long DNA fragments; these fragments can be directly length difference of one nucleotide, and the 3'end nucleotide is radiolabelled with A, T, C, or G. The product was divided into A, T, C, and G, the four electrophoresis lanes; the base can be read in the order to be synthesized, thereby obtaining the DNA sequence to be tested. Thereafter, on the basis of "the Sanger sequencing method," the automatic detection and fluorescence techniques, isotopically labeled with a fluorescent label in place of the four fluorophores, four bases were replaced and automatically detected by imaging techniques, no longer subjected to electrophoresis separately read sequences, greatly improving the speed and accuracy of DNA sequencing. Generation sequencing technology to ensure smooth implementation of Human Genome Project can be obtained secret of human health and disease at the molecular level. However, first-generation sequencing technology has considerable limitations, namely, low throughput, high cost, and long time. Further, since test DNA Sanger sequencing is applied to the support, and cloned in *E. coli* and other bacteria, therefore, it could not be cloned fragments of harmful bacteria, and, in some regions of the genome, such as the centromere and terminal area around the particles is difficult to be cloned, leading to deletion of part of gene sequence. Additionally, the method of analysis is limited ability alleles, SNP detection is very difficult, which facilitates the birth of a new generation of genome sequencing technology.

3.4 Methods detecting SNP

Some technologies such as mass spectrometry, electrophoresis, and microarray hybridization are much more dependent on PCR multiplexing than others to reach their throughput potential [23–25]. However, the efficiency of these technologies was constricted by cross impact in the PCR of primers and DNA samples in one reaction tube. It is evidenced that less than 20 primer pairs could be amplified together that could not support large numbers of SNP measurement. And when multiple SNPs are amplified together in a reaction chamber, only 50–70% SNPs can be amplified successfully, and the amount of products varies greatly from 10 to 1000 folds, what leads to the cooling rate for samples which decreases dramatically—some SNPs that are scored for sample A may not be scored for sample B or C [26–28]. Single-base extension based on multiplexing PCR like mass spectrometry assay is expensive and requires well-trained personnel for performing the various steps of the analysis with a lengthy protocol. For most homogenous detection formats like fluorescence resonance energy transfer and fluorescent polarization, because their testing equipment have very limited capacity of multiplex recently, some technologies such as TaqMan 5′-nuclease assay, DNA hybridization, could not rely on multiplexing PCR to increase their throughput. Genotyping technologies have become a significant bottleneck for these applications despite rapid progress in the field. Exploring fast, accurate, high-throughput SNP genotyping, new technology is particularly urgent. Microfluidics chip is composed of microdroplets, microchannels, and microchambers [29–34]. Each microchamber could be used to amplify only one primer pair. A number of microchambers can be designed to meet the requirement. The physical isolation of different primer pairs is a simple and effective strategy to avoid the drawbacks of conventional multiplex PCR. In order to overcome the SNP genotyping error @ caused by different amplification efficiency, chambers and channels with special structures have also been designed for primer storage and allocation of reaction mixtures. The characteristics of smaller reaction volumes, high-throughput capacity, ease of integration, and portability compared to traditional PCR endow microfluidics (microdroplets, microchannels, and microchambers) with the potential to be a powerful technology to meet SNP genotyping demands. For example, 116-plex PCR designed by Li et al. can be accomplished using a hydrophobically patterned microarray [35]. However, it requires precise operations, and the amplification is performed in an open environment, which risks contamination. Microdroplets (e.g., digital PCR) are also a potential technology for multiplex PCR, but barcoding technology is essential but challenging for multiplex digital PCR. The OpenArray® platform from Applied Biosystems, which was the commercial products for multiplex PCR, is rather expensive and sophisticated, and costly instruments are also required. In brief, these methods for multiplex PCR are effective, but complications in chip processing and/or their high associated costs hinder their wide use.

3.5 Measurement malnutrition-related SNPs and their genotypes

SNP genotype measurement has been widely studied in the risk screen and diagnosis for genetic diseases and chronic diseases, but few studies for nutrient deficiency risk determination. It is agreed that the body micronutrient diagnosis or evaluation is the bottleneck technology barrier since there are numbers of indexes for varieties of micronutrients; in addition, there seems even difficulty to know the genetic information related with micronutrient deficiency. Nutritional genotype studies have facilitated to use MD-SNPs (malnutrition-related SNPs) as risk biomarkers, i.e., vitamins A, D, E, and B_{12}, folate, calcium, iron, zinc, and selenium.

3.5.1 Microfluidic chip designed for malnutrition-related SNPs

Microfluidic chip as high-throughput technology could amplify large numbers of target DNA fragments at the same time in a chip, and the physical isolation of different primer pairs is a simple and effective strategy to avoid the drawbacks of conventional multiplex PCR. Xu et al. took this advantage to reduce the mutual interference and competition among different primers in one tube for multiple PCR [36]. They adopted a modified method with a blocking step, which had showed less contamination than that without blocking method. A study reported by Zhang et al. showed that MD-SNPs were extracted from published studies of GWAS, reviews, and meta-analysis, which epidemically related with micronutrient deficiency, and a method was established by modified microfluidic chip for MD-SNPs measurement by Xu et al. The study would explore possibility to describe MD potential risk from genetic point of view for an individual.

3.5.2 Primer design of nutrition-related SNPs

Primer mix contained three primers, common reverse primer, tailed allele primer 1 and tailed allele primer 2, in a ratio of 5:2:2. Primer mix (0.14 μl, 2 μM for each forward and reverse primers) was preloaded in a reaction chamber. Master mix containing FRET cassette plus enzymes with high-fidelity activity in an optimized buffer solution was stored at −20°C in the refrigerator, kept cool with ice when taken out from refrigerator, and vortex shocked before use (**Figure 1**).

3.5.3 MD-SNP measurement process

The material of the chip was polymethylmethacrylate (PMMA) and was fabricated by machining to final dimensions of 7.5 cm (length) × 2.5 cm (width) × 2 mm (thickness). There were 28 microchambers in a column and 4 parallel columns in a chip that supported for simultaneously testing of 112 SNPs in 3 genotypes of wild type, hybrid type, and mutant type. Each column consisted of a circular inlet and outlet, a "sine-shaped" sample infusing channel, 28 linking channels, and 28 circular reaction chambers. A modified method has been established to prepare the microfluidic chip. Prior to use, the chip was washed with ethanol and ultrapure water and dried with nitrogen gas. Then, the primer pairs were pipetted into different reaction chambers and allowed to dry at room temperature for 30 min. A piece of single-sided, PCR-compatible adhesive tape was used to seal the top side of the chip at 175°C for 1 min. After sealing, the primer-loaded chip was stored at 4°C before use. An aqueous PCR mixture containing PCR master mix and DNA template was loaded into infusing channels by pipetting from the inlets. Outlets and inlets on the bottom side were sealed with adhesive tape to achieve a fully hermetic system. Then, the chip was centrifuged at 4000 rpm for 1 min so that the PCR mixture was uniformly transferred into reaction chambers and thoroughly mixed with the preloaded primers mix, and the final reaction volume was 0.8 μl. Each linking channel was blocked at 150°C for 1 min. Then, the chip was placed on a MasterCycler Nexus flat and pressed with a PMMA block to ensure tight contact and avoid distortion of the chip under high temperature (**Figure 2**).

The temperature program of PCR in the chip was set as follows (**Figure 2**): hot-start activation at 94°C for 15 min, followed by 10 touchdown cycles (94°C for 20 s; touchdown 61–55°C, dropping 0.6°C per cycle), and then followed by 26 cycles of amplification (94°C 20 s; 55°C 60 s). After thermal cycling for 100 min, the amplified products were detected by LuxScan-10 K/A scanner at 40°C or below for

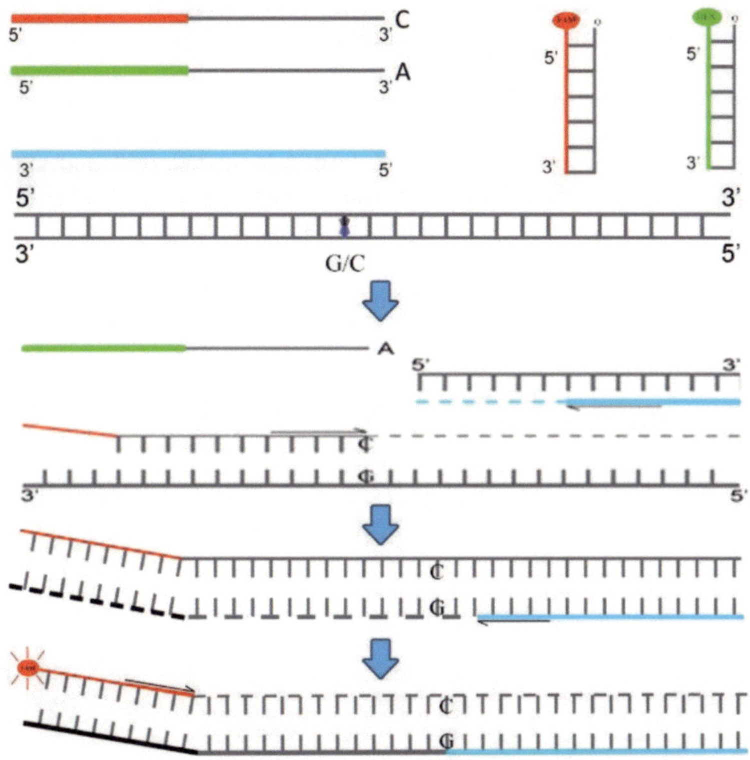

Figure 1.
Steps and principle of allele-specific extension on primer arrays. (A), primer pairs mix containing two different, allele-specific, competing forward primers with unique tail sequences and one reverse primer. Master mix containing FRET cassette plus enzymes with high-fidelity activity in an optimized buffer solution. Test DNA with the SNP of interest. (B), in the first round of PCR, one of the allele-specific primers matches the target SNP and, with the common reverse primer, amplifies the target region; (C), in the second round of PCR, reverse primer binds, elongates, and makes a complement copy of allele-1 tail; (D), in the third round of PCR, FAM-labeled oligo binds to new complementary tail sequence and is no longer quenched; in further rounds of PCR, the levels of allele-specific tail increase. The fluorescent substance-labeled part of the FRET cassette is complementary to new tail sequences and binds, releasing the fluorescent substance from the quencher to generate a fluorescent signal.

15 min. The fluorescence intensity values (FIVs) were used to identify three distinct genotypes of wild type, hybrid type, and mutant type.

3.5.4 Cross-contamination test

Odd-numbered chambers in a column of a chip were preloaded primer mix, while even-numbered chambers were not. In addition, gel electrophoresis was observed with solutions from the corresponding reaction chambers. For specificity of primer mix and accuracy, each primer pair preloaded chamber loaded different template DNAs in a concentration of 10 ng/μl with master mix pipetted into infusing channels. The results were compared with the expected results obtained by next-generation sequencing (NGS). For the selection of appropriate DNA reaction concentration, 52 difficult DNA templates were diluted to 1 ng/μl, 5 ng/μl, 10 ng/μl, and 15 ng/μl to test appropriate DNA reaction concentration, respectively. The repeatability of multiplexed SNPs is observed with four repeats of 52 MD-SNPs in one DNA template. All these experiments were repeated six times. The established method was used to measure DNA templates from six different samples to evaluate the possible MD risk of vitamin A, D, E, and B_{12}, folate, calcium, iron, zinc, and selenium (**Figure 3**).

3.5.5 Multiplex PCR in MD-SNP measurement

Multiplex PCR is a promising method for multiple nucleic acid analysis and detection. Several primers involved in a single tube behaves as multiplex PCR, in which one allele sequence is often preferentially amplified, resulting in the scarcity of other allele sequences, so it is very tedious to establish an optimized multiplex PCR protocol. Most chip-based multiplexed genotyping platforms are suitable for large-scale studies requiring genotypic data with thousands of SNPs. Although

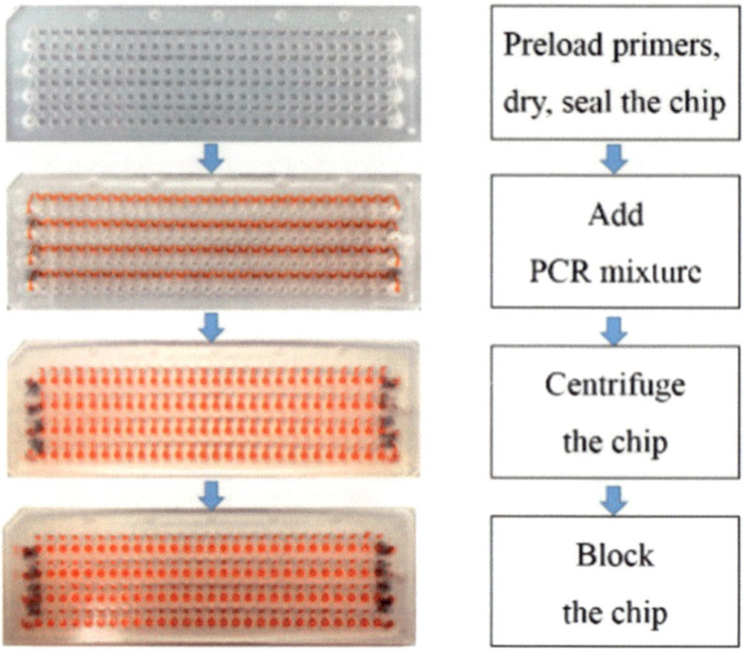

Figure 2.
Workflow protocol of the chip.

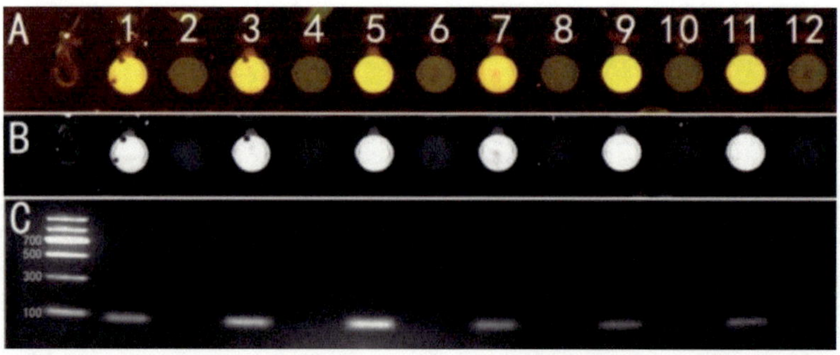

Figure 3.
The cross-contamination testing of adjacent reaction chambers. Odd number and even number represented reaction chambers with and without preloaded primers, respectively. (A) is the fluorescence pseudo-color image; (B) is the corresponding gray scale image; (C) is the electrophoretogram of the amplicons in each reaction chamber which corresponded to the product in the chamber of (A) or (B) above. The lane marked with M represents the DNA marker. The molecular weights of the bands from the top to bottom were 1200, 900, 700, 500, 300, and 100 bps.

multiplexing offers greater throughput with less reagent consumption, it restricts the use which require low to medium marker density, for example, Illumina company requires a minimum number of plates ordered in order to develop specific assays, and this requirement was much higher than individual needs. So Xu et al. developed an innovative microfluidic chip to be the most convenient and cost-effective option for genotyping various individuals, which physically isolates the primer pairs in a reaction chamber. Fifty-two SNPs demonstrated the effectiveness of our strategy by multiplex PCRs and further illustrated its clinical applicability with blood and saliva samples. As a qualitative method, primer pairs of MD-SNPs designed in this study could be successfully amplified in the given conditions and replicated target DNA fragments with additional florescence carriers of FAM and HEX. Three genotypes of mutant type, hybrid type, and wild type could be identified specifically and accurately by the measurement. The sample chambers showed averagely at least two times higher FIV than that of NTCs. 5 ng/μl or higher suggested the suitable DNA concentration for the selected 52 MD-SNPs, although the optimal concentration for each primer pair may be different. The method showed high repeatability in both inner chips and among chips. The results of 52 MD-SNPs determined by MD-chips and NGS were completely the same, suggesting a high accuracy of the method.

There are several advantages of the microfluidic chip multiplex PCR: (1) the generality of the primer design principle which was adopted by this microfluidic chip assays. The principle is developed for common use in all genotyping assays to stringently target the two alleles with standard PCR conditions and similar amplification efficiencies and significantly decreases the cost in PCR reagents and labors. (2) It is more specific. The microfluidic chip genotyping results were completely coincident with next-generation sequencing results. (3) It is easier. All the primer pairs are physically isolated; deleting or adding one or a few primer pairs from a multiplex PCR primer panel will not alter the performance of the other primer pairs with standard PCR conditions; almost no additional optimization is required. So, the universal protocol is viable for developing diverse multiplex PCR applications. (4) Its throughput is flexible. The selection of a technique has to weigh factors of instrument, throughput, technical support, and cost. Because of its unprecedented specificity, simplicity, and flexibility of throughout, the chip could serve as a powerful tool in clinical individual nutriment deficiency risk diagnostics for multiplexed detection of nutriments. The results of the analysis performed using the chip may provide early and crucial information for physicians to prevent nutriment deficiency risk and conduct appropriate nutritional intervention.

4. Malnutrition risk evaluated by personal SNPs

4.1 Expression of malnutrition risk with MD-SNPs

The MD-SNP chip method was used to measure MD risk of six students which showed distinguished differences of genetic potentials. The MD risk of six students was shown in a colored image in a pattern of SNP genotypes in three colors. The wild type was in red, hybrid type in orange, and mutant type in green. The risk of individuals in a micronutrient deficiency could be identified by the differences of red color areas. The genotype for each SNP of micronutrients in a person could be presented with the image (**Figure 4**).

4.2 Guiding on nutrient intake with MD-SNP

The combination of this method with present laboratory measurement might comprehensively explain individual MD risk in both genetic and diet environmental

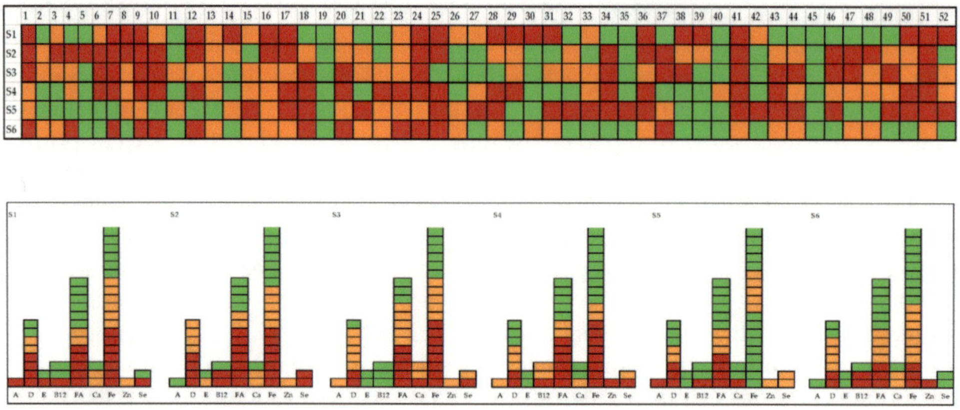

Figure 4.
The color grade of nine MD-SNPs in six measured individual samples. S, sample.

conditions, thus facilitating with precise nutrition intervention. For example, MTHFR-C677T polymorphism has been extensively studied, and the association between the TT genotype and low folate status is well documented. Individuals with the TT genotype seem to be particularly susceptible to insufficient status of several B vitamins, and they may need to consume more folate to maintain serum folate levels similar to those found in individuals with the CC/CT genotypes. A study by Crider et al. reported that daily 0.8 mg folic acid may be necessary to lower homocysteine concentration for Chinese hypertensive subjects with CT or TT genotype, which have important clinical and public health implications [37]. The Centers for Disease Control and Prevention in the United States showed in 1992 that women who have previously suffered a NTD-affected pregnancy are advised to take 4 mg of folic acid daily before conception and during the first months of pregnancy [38]. Then we could calculate the required amount of an individual micronutrients according to SNPs.

In the real world, the body's nutritional status is regulated by multiple genes and nutrients. For example, homocysteine (Hcy) is a precursor of methionine and cysteine. Methionine converts into S-adenosyl methionine, which acts as a universal methyl donor. These multistep reactions involve various enzymes and cofactors in the form of essential micronutrients, which include vitamin B complex family (B_2, B_6, B_9, and B_{12}). Therefore, in measuring tHcy, folic acid and vitamin B_{12}, vis-a`-vis the genotypes of the Hcy-pathway genes, Zhang et al. evaluated contribution of the individual variables (SNPs of Hcy-pathway genes) in the development of the phenotype (Hcy level) and get an estimate of the relative contribution of the environment (vitamins) in modulating the effect of genotypes in this region. Hyperhomocysteinemia is a result of either reduced enzymatic activity in the enzymes that participate in homocysteine metabolism and/or a reduction in the concentrations of plasma B vitamins, particularly, folate. Dietary intake of folate or folic acid supplementation can lower the concentration of p-tHcy. The establishment of gender and age as covariates is associated with SNP HCY polygenic risk score model (PRS), PRS = −0.024802rs2274976 + 0.025011rs1801131 + 0.205567rs1801133–0.025646rs1805087–0.025047rs2118981 + 0.340703rs492602–0.448651rs602662 + 0.067954sex + 0.060073 age+1.553543; sex, female 0, male 1; age, Year ($R^2 = 0.4084$, $p < 2.2e\text{-}16$).

The incidence of early detection, prevention, and intervention was the fundamental goal of promoting human health; predicting the probability of an individual assessment of the risk of susceptibility to disease was the core clinical decision-making, especially for the detection and prevention of common diseases. The current clinical data for common adult disease risk often relied on basic human indicators, such as age, gender and ethnicity, lifestyle, and basic health indicators, such as body mass index, smoking status, alcohol use, and physical activity habits; suffering disease relevant to the biomarkers like blood pressure level and biochemical indexes; analysis of environmental exposure, such as air pollution, heavy metals, and other environmental toxins; and family history. Many recent studies have begun to demonstrate the utility of gene association analysis and access to individual genetic susceptibility to a disease useful for the guidance of information from the probability of large population data. In theory, gene mapping could be considered a useful part of a healthy management.

Author details

Junsheng Huo* and Chunhong Zhang
Institute of Nutrition and Health of China's Center for Disease Control and Prevention, China

*Address all correspondence to: huojs@ninh.chinacdc.cn

References

[1] Soeters P, Bozzetti F, Cynober L, Forbes A, Shenkin A, Sobotka L. Defining malnutrition: A plea to rethink. Clinical Nutrition. 2016;**S0261-5614**(16):31272-31279. DOI: 10.1016/j.clnu.2016.09.032

[2] Draft of the Rome Declaration on Nutrition. https://www.who.int/nutrition/events/icn2_draft_RomeDeclaration_Nutrition_en.pdf

[3] Initiatives D. 2018 Global Nutrition Report: Shining a Light to Spur Action on Nutrition. Bristol, UK: Development Initiatives; 2018

[4] Yang YX, Ge KY. Encyclopedia of Nutrition Science. Beijing: People's medical publishing house; 2019

[5] Haugen AC, Schug TT, Collman G, Heinder JJ. Evolution of DOHaD: The impact of environmental health sciences. Journal of Developmental Origins of Health and Disease. 2015;**6**(2):55-64. DOI: 10.1017/s2040174414000580

[6] McLaren Christine E, Stela ML, Garner Chad P, et al. Associations between single nucleotide polymorphisms in iron-related genes and iron status in multiethnic populations. PLoS One. 2012;7(6):e38339

[7] Smithells RW, Chinn ER. Meclozine and Fetal malformations: A prospective study. British Medical Journal. 1964;**1**(5377):217-218

[8] Frosst P, Blom HJ, Milos R, et al. A candidate genetic risk factor for vascular disease: A common mutation in methylenetetrahydrofolate reductase. Nature Genetics. 1995;**10**(1):111-113

[9] Chunhong Z, Junsheng H, Jing S, et al. The association of maternal MTR and MTRR polymorphisms with neural tube defect of offspring: Meta-analysis. The Journal of Chinese Preventive Medicine. 2018;**19**:726-733 (In Chinese)

[10] Chunhong Z, Junsheng H, Jing S, et al. Meta-analysis on relationship between the Chinese maternal MTHFR gene polymorphism (C677T) and neural tube defects in offspring. The Journal of Hygiene Research. 2018;**47**:312-317 (In Chinese)

[11] Daniel C, Kevin D, Noah S, et al. A cross-sectional study of dietary and genetic predictors of blood Folate levels in healthy young adults. Nutrients. 2017;**9**(9):994

[12] Wilcken B. Geographical and ethnic variation of the 677C>T allele of 5,10 methylene tetrahydrofolate reductase (MTHFR): Findings from over 7000 newborns from 16 areas worldwide. Journal of Medical Genetics. 2003;**40**(8):619-625

[13] Clifford AJ, Chen K, McWade L, et al. Gender and single nucleotide polymorphisms in MTHFR, BHMT, SPTLC1, CRBP2, CETP, and SCARB1 are significant predictors of plasma homocysteine normalized by RBC folate in healthy adults. The Journal of Nutrition. 2012;**142**:1764-1771

[14] Jacobsen N. LNA-enhanced detection of single nucleotide polymorphisms in the apolipoprotein E. Nucleic Acids Research. 2002;**30**:100e-1100e

[15] Major JM, Yu K, Chung CC, et al. Genome-wide association study identifies three common variants associated with serologic response to vitamin E supplementation in men. The Journal of Nutrition. 2012;**142**:866-871

[16] O'Seaghdha CM, Wu H, Yang Q, et al. Meta-analysis of genome-wide association studies identifies six new

loci for serum calcium concentrations. PLoS Genetics. 2013;**9**:e1003796

[17] McLaren CE, McLachlan S, Garner CP, et al. Associations between single nucleotide polymorphisms in iron-related genes and iron status in multiethnic populations. PLoS One. 2012;**7**:e38339

[18] Fredriksen A, Meyer K, Ueland PM, et al. Large-scale population-based metabolic phenotyping of thirteen genetic polymorphisms related to one-carbon metabolism. Human Mutation. 2007;**28**:856-865

[19] Li WX, Dai SX, Zheng JJ, et al. Homocysteine metabolism gene polymorphisms (MTHFR C677T, MTHFR A1298C, MTR A2756G and MTRR A66G) jointly elevate the risk of folate deficiency. Nutrients. 2015;**7**:6670-6687

[20] Liang S, Zhou Y, Wang H, et al. The effect of multiple single nucleotide polymorphisms in the folic acid pathway genes on homocysteine metabolism. BioMed Research International. 2014;**2014**:560183

[21] Tanaka T, Scheet P, Giusti B, et al. Genome-wide association study of vitamin B6, vitamin B12, folate, and homocysteine blood concentrations. American Journal of Human Genetics. 2009;**84**:477-482

[22] Ahn J, Yu K, Stolzenberg-Solomon R, et al. Genome-wide association study of circulating vitamin D levels. Human Molecular Genetics. 2010;**19**:2739-2745

[23] Steluti J, Carvalho AM, Carioca AAF, et al. Genetic variants involved in one-carbon metabolism: Polymorphism frequencies and differences in homocysteine concentrations in the folic acid fortification era. Nutrients. 2017;**9**:539-550

[24] Sexton TR, Henry RJ, McManus LJ, et al. Capture of assay template by multiplex PCR of long amplicons for genotyping SNPs and indels with MALDI-TOF mass spectrometry. Molecular Breeding. 2009;**25**:471-480

[25] Tajadini M, Panjehpour M, Javanmard SH. Comparison of SYBR green and Taqman methods in quantitative real-time polymerase chain reaction analysis of four adenosine receptor subtypes. Advances in Biology Research. 2014;**3**:85

[26] Fan JB, Oliphant A, Shen R, et al. Highly parallel SNP genotyping. Cold Spring Harbor Symposia on Quantitative Biology. 2003;**68**:69

[27] Hindson BJ, Ness KD, Masquelier DA, et al. High-throughput droplet digital PCR system for absolute quantitation of DNA copy number. Analytical Chemistry. 2011;**83**:8604-8610

[28] Morrison T, Hurley J, Garcia J, et al. Nanoliter high throughput quantitative PCR. Nucleic Acids Research. 2006;**34**:e123

[29] Shen F, Du W, Davydova EK, et al. Nanoliter multiplex PCR arrays on a slipChip. Analytical Chemistry. 2010;**82**:4606-4612

[30] Chen X, Sullivan PF. Single nucleotide polymorphism genotyping: Biochemistry, protocol, cost and throughput. The Pharmacogenomics Journal. 2003;**3**:77-96

[31] Sundberg SO, Wittwer CT, Chao G, et al. Spinning disk platform for microfluidic digital polymerase chain reaction. Analytical Chemistry. 2010;**82**:1546-1550

[32] Tomi Pastinen MR, Lindroos K, Tainola P, et al. A system for specific, high-throughput genotyping by

allele-specific primer extension on microarrays. Genome Research. 2000;**10**:1031-1042

[33] Yan H, Zhu Y, Zhang Y, et al. Multiplex detection of bacteria on an integrated centrifugal disk using bead-beating lysis and loop-mediated amplification. Scientific Reports. 2017;7:1-12

[34] Palani K, Chaoyong James Y, Cronier SA, et al. High-throughput single copy DNA amplification and cell analysis in engineered Nanoliter droplets. Analytical Chemistry. 2008;**80**:3522-3529

[35] Li Y, Guo SJ, Shao N, Tu S, et al. A universal multiplex PCR strategy for 100-plex amplification using a hydrophobically patterned microarray. Lab on a Chip. 2011;**11**:3609-3618

[36] Xu Y, Yan H, Zhang Y, et al. A fully sealed plastic chip for multiplex PCR and its application in bacteria identification. Lab on a Chip. 2015;**15**:2826-2834

[37] Crider KS, Zhu JH, Hao L, et al. MTHFR 677C->T genotype is associated with folate and homocysteine concentrations in a large, population-based, double-blind trial of folic acid supplementation. American Journal of Clinical Nutrition. 2011;**93**(6):1365-1372

[38] CDC (Centers for Disease Control and Prevention). Recommendations for the use of folic acid to reduce the number of cases of spina bifida and other neural tube defects. MMWR. Morbidity and Mortality Weekly Report. 1992;**41**(RR-14):001